Nature's Nutrition

A Comprehensive Resource Guide for Super Foods, Natural Supplements and Preventative Health

Rory M. Celmin

Executive Editor: Ginny Greene

Cover Design: Alan Karalian

Contact info:
email: RMCBooks@yahoo.com
website: https://www.createspace.com/3692862
twitter: @VitalityHealth9

ISBN-13: 978-0-9840186-1-1
ISBN-10: 0984018611

Legal Disclaimer: This book is intended for informational purposes only, is not meant to replace the advice or consultation of a doctor or physician and should not be construed as personal medical advice. Readers should always consult appropriate health professionals for any matters relating to their health and well being. Neither the author nor publisher is advocating, offering or participating in any health treatment, professional advice or services to the reader, nor will they be responsible for any adverse effects, damage, injury, loss or consequences allegedly arising from any information, suggestions or recommendations in this book. Readers who fail to consult appropriate health professionals assume the risk of any injuries. Know your allergies and always consult your doctor/physician before consuming unfamiliar foods or supplements.

If we could give every individual the right amount of nourishment and exercise, not too little and not too much, we would have found the safest way to health.

~ Hippocrates ~

TABLE OF CONTENTS

Part One: The Fundamentals of Nutrition

Part Two: Super Foods, Natural Supplements, Therapeutic Spices, Holistic Herbs

Part Three: Personal Health and Nutrition

Part Four: Common Health Disorders

Part Five: Appendix

Part One

The Fundamentals of Nutrition

~ Preventative Health ~

I have always been intrigued at how nature provides us with all the nutrients we need to stay healthy. Balanced nutrition is the key to optimizing health, and is done by consuming foods from a wide variety of sources. It allows us to function at our fullest potential, and is often the link between diet and cancer prevention. Minerals are one of the basic foundations of health, but over-farming and unsustainable farming practices have left soils depleted and many people in our society mineral deficient. Nutritional deficiencies are believed to be the root of many degenerative health disorders, and may be prevented or corrected by proper nutrition because the body is a self-healing organism and conditions often improve. For example, liver and lung tissues regenerate, skin replenishes and rebuilds and the body sweats when we have a fever. These are signs the human body wants to fix itself.

The modern day American diet is loaded with sodium, sugar, white flour, fried foods, hydrogenated oils and saturated fats that starve the body of essential nutrients it needs to function properly. These foods destroy enzyme production and inhibit proper digestive functions, making it difficult for the body to eliminate harmful substances. When toxins accumulate in the kidneys, liver and other major organs, they slow down bodily functions which usually results in a lack of energy, limited mental clarity and may sometimes lead to depression. Food discipline and breaking bad eating habits is essential for maximizing health and well-being. Taking a natural, preventative approach to nutrition has helped many people feel healthier and more energetic, which also gives them the motivation to continue.

The main factors that influence health and longevity are genetics, environment, lifestyle and diet. Being proactive about staying healthy includes eating low-fat, high-fiber, nutrient-dense foods, drinking plenty of water, getting proper sleep, and about 30 minutes of cardiovascular exercise each day. Paying attention to what you eat and learning how your body benefits or reacts to certain foods is crucial in knowing how nutrition relates specifically to you. Moreover, since health care costs are going through the roof, it is important to have affordable, wholesome food options that are beneficial for improving and maintaining health.

Preventative health should be a dietary priority for everyone, and may be the solution for many common health disorders. We all know that apples are good for us. But what if a smoker learns that apples help improve lung function because the pectin they contain binds to carcinogens from cigarette smoke and helps eliminate them from the body? This is the kind of relevant information that is needed to promote preventative health, and can help people better understand their own specific nutritional needs…*just some food for thought.*

~ Evolution of Nutrition ~

The importance of nutrition has been studied and well respected since the dawn of civilization. The rise in agriculture, also known as the "Neolithic Revolution," began around 10000 B.C. and marked the transition from hunting and gathering to agriculture, communities and settlement. No longer did hunters have to follow the migration of animal herds – they had locally grown foods to survive on. They were now able to produce various fruits and vegetables including almonds, apples, cherries, dates, lentils, maize, and such grains as millet, rice and wheat. Between 6500 B.C. and 3200 B.C., livestock such as cattle, chickens, goats, pigs and sheep were domesticated in Asia, Greece and parts of the Middle East. The advancement of agriculture led to the construction of permanent cities, which eventually led to the establishment of large civilizations.

One of the birthplaces of agriculture is along the fertile grounds of the Nile River where the ancient Egyptians established their prosperous civilization. Bread and beer were abundant staples of the Egyptian diet, and also included various vegetables, fruits, fish and fowl. The Egyptians understood the synergy between food and health, and based their nutrition system on the sun. They believed we embody the sun's light energy from the foods we consume. This light energy circulating in our bodies, called "radiance," is believed to be the life force of all living creatures. Levels of radiance in the body were affected by certain foods and were believed to influence physical balance, proper growth, aging and overall health. Fruits and vegetables were high-radiance foods and were consumed in abundance, whereas dairy was a low-radiance food and was consumed far less.

Other ancient civilizations - the Chinese and the Greeks - were also very familiar with the healing properties of food. Traditional Chinese Medicine, or TCM, dates back to around 5000 B.C. and focuses on harmony with nature and energy flow. Along with acupuncture and massage, TCM's extensive use of nutrition and herbs to treat a myriad of ailments including digestive, cardiovascular, respiratory, skin and inflammatory disorders is well documented. The ancient Greeks helped form the foundation of modern medicine with the remarkable work of Hippocrates. Revered as the greatest physician of his time, he was able to accurately describe symptoms of disease such as pneumonia and epilepsy, and believed that the body must be treated as a whole, not as individual parts. Hippocrates also believed that optimal health comes from proper foods as well as fresh air, cleanliness and adequate rest. Also known as the "Father of Modern Medicine," Hippocrates is famous for his quote, "*let food be your medicine and medicine be your food.*" As more food items became available throughout the centuries, the relationship between nutrition and health became more apparent.

Some anthropological evidence suggests that an increase in the consumption of animal foods was associated with stimulating brain growth. The brains of our early ancestors became more advanced and began to grow in size around the same time butchered animal bones and stone tools were found. The result was improved hunting and gathering skills which enabled these ancient tribes to collect and consume larger quantities of higher quality, nutrient-rich foods. This eventually led to further brain development and more advanced social behavior which increased their overall chances of survival. Although we now know that plant-based foods provide more nutrients and are associated with a lower risk of degenerative diseases, meat consumption seemed to be a contributing factor to the success of human evolution.

With this in mind, did the human body evolve to consume an herbivore, carnivore or omnivore diet? The human gastrointestinal tract is approximately 25 feet long and is able to digest both animal and plant foods. However, some evidence suggests the human body was designed primarily for plant foods. Humans have 20 molars for crushing and grinding plant foods, eight incisors for biting into fruits and vegetables, and only four canine teeth that are designed for eating meat. Our jaws move both vertically to tear meat and laterally to crush plant foods, whereas a carnivore's jaw only moves vertically. Additional evidence indicating the similarity between herbivores and humans is the length of our digestive system. Carnivores have short intestinal tracts ideal for digesting meats, whereas humans and herbivores both have long intestinal tracts that are better suited for digesting plant foods.

Most of the discoveries in the field of nutrition have taken place during the 20th century. This era, known as the "Golden Age of Nutrition," is when most of the macro- and micronutrients were identified and nutritional requirements were established. During the 1920s & 1930s, Dr. Weston A. Price, a pioneering dentist from Cleveland and author of *Nutrition & Physical Degeneration,* conducted extensive research studying dental and nutritional health of various remote civilizations. He traveled throughout the world comparing health conditions among a long list of isolated and more modernized cultures including African tribes of Kenya, Tanzania and Uganda, Alaskan Inuit tribes, Australian Aborigines, New Zealand Maori, the Gaelic Highlands of Scotland, remote Swiss villages, Indians of the Amazon and ancient civilizations of Peru. Dr. Price examined and documented many dental, facial, skull and bone growth deformities in relation to nutritional deficiencies. He concluded that isolated, less modernized cultures consumed more nutrient-dense foods and had superior physical and dental health compared to more modernized civilizations. Dr. Price also believed that fat-soluble vitamins (A, D, E & K) were especially important for optimizing health and acted as catalysts for proper nutrient absorption.

Denis Burkitt, M.D., and Hugh Trowel, M.D., editors of *Western Diseases: Their Emergence and Prevention*, continued the monumental work of Dr. Price by further examining primitive cultures and their varying rates of disease. They were able to compare epidemiological data of primitive and modernizing cultures, their lifestyle differences and changes in dietary habits dating back 400 generations to the emergence of agriculture. Burkitt and Trowel concluded that maintaining traditional diets of wholesome, unprocessed plant foods and lean protein resulted in extremely low rates of degenerative diseases. As certain cultures began to deviate from their traditional foods and consume a modernized Western diet, there was a sharp increase of digestive disorders and obesity. As they continued to shift away from plant-based foods and consume meats higher in saturated fat, conditions such as arthritis, diabetes, cardiovascular disease, high blood pressure and cancer became much more common.

Today the American diet consists of more canned, processed, microwaveable and fast foods which are far less nutritious but have become commonplace. These foods are usually higher in sodium, sugar, white flour, saturated fats and hydrogenated vegetable oils which are all linked to an increased risk of many health disorders. Additionally, the modern-day domestication of farm animals has led to injections of growth hormones, much higher levels of saturated fat and scarce amounts of omega 3's compared to their free-range counterparts of the past. Our ancestors had much lower rates of degenerative diseases because their diet consisted almost entirely of organic, nutrient-dense plant foods and lean, free-range livestock rich in omega 3's.

In the United States, over a billion pounds of poisonous herbicides and pesticides are sprayed on our food crops every year. Even though they are somewhat effective for their intended purpose, most of these powerful chemicals are absorbed into the air, soil and our water supply which eventually leaches into our food supply. The Price-Pottenger Nutrition Foundation (PPNF) has preserved Dr. Price's trailblazing research and also archives the work of other nutritional pioneers. PPNF advocates humane animal husbandry, encourages soil improvement and promotes organic farming and gardening practices. This includes non-toxic, pollution-free housing, holistic medical therapies and natural, wholesome food choices for livestock. PPNF contends that primitive, non-modernized diets contained more nutrients than our Western diet, and that modern man must incorporate the nutrition fundamentals of our ancestors to maximize our health potential.

Organic farming increases the nutritional content of food, and will help slow the toxic trend of chemical additives. Not only does it provide more minerals, but it also improves soil quality, increases crop tolerance to drought and protects the ecosystem by encouraging diverse plant and wildlife. Organic certification is the public's assurance that products have been grown and handled in accordance with national organic standards. U.S. farmers are turning to certified organic farming systems as a way to lower costs, decrease reliance on nonrenewable resources, capture high-value markets and premium prices, and boost farm income. Organic farming utilizes ecologically based practices such as cultural and biological pest management, and excludes all antibiotics, hormones and synthetic chemicals from food crops and livestock production to ensure organic integrity. Since the early 1990s, organic farming has been one of the fastest growing segments of agriculture in the United States. Sales of organic foods have increased each year by approximately 20%, reaching nearly $24 billion by 2010. The demand for organic foods will forever grow, and its significance to our health and longevity has never been greater.

~ Elements of Nutrition ~

Amino Acids

Amino acids are the building blocks that form proteins, the end products of protein digestion and are necessary in the chemical processes that create life. They are what make up muscles, tendons, ligaments, organs, glands, hair, nails and body fluids. Amino acids contain carbon, hydrogen, nitrogen and oxygen and help maintain a healthy pH level in the body. They are responsible for exchanging nutrients between blood, tissues and lymph and are part of the chromosome structure through which genetic codes are transferred from parent to child. Amino acids assist the metabolic process, enabling vitamins and minerals to function properly. They also protect against allergies and autoimmune disorders, and as neurotransmitters they are vital for the transmission of nerve impulses from the brain to the cells. Most amino acids can be manufactured by the human body, but there are nine essential amino acids that cannot be produced by the body so they need to be obtained from food sources. Foods rich in amino acids include almonds, barley, beans, beef, brewer's yeast, brown rice, buckwheat, chicken, dairy, eggs, fish, liver, nuts/seeds, oatmeal, quinoa, soy foods, turkey and wheat. The essential amino acids include histidine, isoleucine, leucine, lysine, methionine, phenylalanine, threonine, tryptophan and valine. Nonessential amino acids include alanine, arginine, asparagine, cysteine, glutamine, glutathione, glycine, proline, serine, taurine and tyrosine.

Antioxidants

Antioxidants are organic substances that help protect the body from toxins, and are among the most important components of staying healthy. Free radicals are formed from ingesting toxins from certain foods, exposure to air pollution, cigarette smoke, radiation, agricultural chemicals, cleaners and even tap water. In many cases, toxins may increase the risk of cancer, cardiovascular disease and premature aging. Antioxidants synergistically work together to neutralize free radicals and protect the body so smaller doses of various antioxidants can be more effective. They are beneficial for easing arthritis and inflammation, protecting against atherosclerosis and strengthening the immune system. Antioxidants are helpful for slowing the aging process, improving skin quality and blocking the effects of sun damage on the skin. Due to their powerful oxidative properties, they are also known to be beneficial for senility and Alzheimer's disease, and promote eye health by lower the risk of macular degeneration. Antioxidant food sources include apples, artichokes, beans, beets, bell peppers, berries, broccoli, carrots, garlic, grapes (red), green tea, kale, oregano, pecans, prunes, soy foods, spinach, sweet potatoes, tomatoes, turmeric and whole grains. Cancer-fighting antioxidants include carotenoids (lutein, lycopene), flavonoids (resveratrol, quercitin) CoQ10, selenium and vitamins A, C, E and zinc.

Enzymes

Enzymes are protein molecules that act as catalysts and play a vital role in all biochemical and bodily functions. They help breakdown sugars, starches, proteins and fats and are necessary for nutrient absorption, proper digestion and normalizing metabolism. Enzymes generate energy on the cellular level, stimulate brain function and help repair damaged organs, tissues and cells. They are responsible for maintaining iron levels in the blood, and stopping wounds from bleeding by helping blood to coagulate. Enzymes are also beneficial for improving respiratory health, alleviating food allergies and reducing yeast infections. Additional benefits include easing arthritis and lower back pain, and protecting against digestive disorders such as heartburn, indigestion and Crohn's disease. These life-sustaining enzymes are found in raw fruits and vegetables including apples, avocados, bananas, beans, mangoes, papayas, pineapples, sprouts and whole grains. Enzymes include amylase, bromelain, cellulase, chymopapain, diastase, glucoamylase, hemicellulase, hyaluronidase, invertase, lactase, lipase, maltase, pancreatin, papain, pectinase, pepsin, phytase, plasmin, protease, rennin and trypsin.

Fatty Acids

Omega 3, 6 and 9 fatty acids are organic compounds of carbon chains that are the building blocks of fats and are needed to maintain proper health. Originally classified as vitamin F, the omega 3 and omega 6 fatty acids are "essential" because the body needs them but cannot produce them on its own. Omega 3's are associated with additional health benefits due to their content of fatty acids *docosahexaenoic acid* (DHA) and *eicosapentaenoic acid* (EPA). Not only does DHA improve cardiovascular function, it is a vital constituent of the brain making up about 8% of the brain's weight. EPA is essential for blood clotting, stimulating brain and nerve function and helps lower cholesterol and triglyceride levels. Consuming an equal amount of omega 3's as omega 6's is a healthy goal to strive for. Western diets have a considerable amount more of omega 6's than omega 3's, and this imbalance is believed to increase the risk of autoimmune and inflammatory disorders, cardiovascular disease, senility and depression. Food sources for omega 3's include wild-caught salmon, herring, mackerel, flaxseed oil and leafy green vegetables. These foods contain powerful anti-aging properties and are beneficial for reducing the risk of cancer and diabetes, alleviating arthritis and inflammation and improving brain function. Omega 6 foods include almonds, avocados, cereals, chicken, eggs, legumes, nuts, pumpkin seeds, turkey and vegetable oils (canola, corn, cottonseed, flaxseed, safflower, soybean, sunflower and wheat germ). These are needed in smaller amounts and are associated with lowering cholesterol levels and improving cardiovascular function. Olive oil is the best source of omega 9's, but they can also be found in foods like almonds, avocados, cashews, olives, peanuts, pecans, pistachios and sesame oil. Omega 9 fatty acids improve cardiovascular health, protect against atherosclerosis, lower cholesterol levels, reduce the risk of cancer, strengthen the immune system and help control blood sugar levels.

Fiber

Also known as *bulk* or *roughage*, dietary fibers are the indigestible parts of plant food that pass unchanged through the stomach, intestine and colon. They are known to provide many health benefits such as helping to reduce the risk of colon cancer, constipation, diabetes, cardiovascular disease and high blood pressure while increasing energy and promoting weight loss. Fiber is categorized into two categories: soluble fiber (dissolves in water) and insoluble fiber (does not dissolve in water). Soluble fiber controls blood sugar and cholesterol levels, and are found in apples, barley, beans, carrots, citrus fruits, flaxseed, oats, oranges, psyllium, raisins, soybeans and strawberries. Insoluble fiber helps alleviate constipation and normalize digestion, and is found in foods like cauliflower, corn bran, fruit skins, green beans, nuts/seeds, leafy green vegetables and whole grains.

Phytonutrients

Phytonutrients are organic, biologically active substances found in nearly all plants (fruits, vegetables, grains, legumes) that are rich in antioxidants and come in a full spectrum of health-promoting colors. They are rich in dietary fiber, enzymes and vitamin-like substances that offer powerful protection against cancer, cardiovascular disease, atherosclerosis and many other degenerative disorders. Phytonutrients are also associated with inhibiting the growth of tumors, reducing ulcers, protecting against diabetes, helping to lower blood pressure and cholesterol levels and improving cardiovascular health. Additional benefits of these natural compounds include strengthening the immune system, improving lung health, and protecting against various forms of dementia like senility and Alzheimer's disease. Phytonutrients also contain anti-inflammatory properties that help alleviate arthritis and provide natural pain relief. Food sources of these life-extending nutrients include apricots, beets, bell peppers, berries, broccoli, cabbage, cantaloupe, carrots, celery, collard greens, garlic, grapefruit, grapes (red), green tea, lemons/limes, nectarines, onions, papayas, pineapples, soy foods, spinach, sweet potatoes, tomatoes and watermelon.

~ Macronutrients ~

Carbohydrates

Carbohydrates are the primary source of energy the body needs to function properly. They supply blood glucose that fuels the brain and keeps red blood cells healthy. There are two types of carbohydrates to be familiar with: simple and complex. Simple carbohydrates are composed of either one sugar molecule (monosaccharides) or two sugar molecules (disaccharides). Glucose and fructose (fruit sugar) are monosaccharides whereas sucrose (table sugar), lactose (milk sugar) and maltose (malt sugar) are disaccharides. Complex carbohydrates are composed of multiple sugar molecules that form longer, more complex chains. These are the most nutritious source of carbohydrates and include vegetables, fruits, beans, nuts, seeds and whole grains (amaranth, barley, brown rice, buckwheat, millet, oats, quinoa, spelt, wheat, wild rice). They provide dietary fiber, vitamins, minerals and other important nutrients that help protect the body from a number of health disorders. Another important aspect of carbohydrates to understand, especially for diabetics, is the glycemic index (GI). This is a measure of how fast carbohydrates will absorb into the blood stream and raise blood sugar levels. Avoid processed foods like candy, chips, desserts and soda; they lack nutritional content and are high in calories. The following table lists the various types of carbohydrates and their food sources.

Carbohydrates

Simple Carbohydrates	Food Sources	Complex Carbohydrates	Food Sources
Monosaccharides (1 sugar molecule)		**Polysaccharides (chains of sugar molecules)**	
Glucose	fruits, honey, sweet corn, root vegetables	Vegetables	bell peppers, broccoli, cabbage, carrots, celery, onions, spinach, sweet potatoes, tomatoes
Fructose	fruits, honey, maple syrup	Fruits	apples, bananas, berries, grapes, grapefruit, melons, oranges, peaches, pears, plums, raisins
Disaccharides (2 sugar molecules)		Legumes	beans, lentils
Sucrose	table sugar, processed foods	Whole Grains	amaranth, barley, bran, brown rice, buckwheat, cornmeal, millet, muesli, oats, quinoa, wheat germ
Maltose	barley malt syrup, malted grain products	Nuts/Seeds	almonds, cashews, flaxseeds, peanuts, pistachios, pumpkin seeds, sunflower seeds, walnuts
Lactose	milk		

Fats

Despite the American obesity epidemic due to excessive fat consumption, fat is an important source of energy for the body that supports growth and is necessary for proper brain development of a child. It is beneficial for hormone health, regulating metabolism and is the primary structural component of cellular membranes. There are three types of dietary fats: *saturated, monounsaturated and polyunsaturated.* Saturated fats are generally from animal products like cheese, cream and milk, as well as fatty meats like beef, ham, lamb and pork. Excessive amounts may raise cholesterol levels and increase the risk of heart attack and stroke. Monounsaturated fats are the "good fats" that help reduce the risk of cardiovascular disease, lower cholesterol levels, alleviate arthritis and promote weight loss. They are found in vegetables, avocados, nuts and seeds as well as canola oil and olive oil. Polyunsaturated fats are also considered "good fats" and include corn, cottonseed, safflower, soybean, sunflower oils and walnuts. However, they are high in calories, and excessive consumption may increase the risk of cardiovascular disease. The USDA recommends no more than 30% of total daily calories come from fat, and no more than 10% come from unsaturated fats. The following table is a listing of common foods categorized by their percentage of calories from fat.

Food Sources	% of Calories from Fat
butter, chocolate, cream, cream cheese, Italian dressing, macadamia nuts, mayonnaise, olives, pecans	90 - 100%
avocado, bacon, beef brisket, coconut, egg yolks, hot dogs, ribs, sausage, sour cream, steak	80 - 90%
almonds, cashews, cheese (blue, cheddar, Swiss), half & half, lamb chops, lobster, luncheon meats, peanut butter, pumpkin seeds, salami, sesame seeds, sunflower seeds, walnuts	70 - 80%
beef (lean), cheese (mozzarella, ricotta), eggs (whole), ham, lamb (lean), tuna fish (in oil)	60 - 70%
anchovies, chicken (dark meat), chuck steak (lean), herring, mackerel, sea bass	50 - 60%
chili, crackers, granola, halibut, ice cream (low-fat), salmon, sardines, tofu, turkey, whole milk, yogurt	40 - 50%
cottage cheese, milk (low-fat), soybeans, yogurt	30 - 40%
chicken (white meat), chicken noodle soup, turkey breast	20 - 30%
cottage cheese (low-fat), garbanzo beans, grapes, kale, lettuce, mustard greens, oatmeal, strawberries, turnip greens	10 - 20%
apples, asparagus, blueberries, buckwheat, cabbage, cauliflower, celery, chestnuts, cucumber, eggplant, lemons, melons, mushrooms, raisins, rye, zucchini	5 - 10%
artichokes, barley, beans (kidney, lima), brown rice, carrots, egg whites, fruits/vegetables (most), onions, pasta, peas, potatoes, raisins, skim milk, whole grains	0 - 5%

Protein

Proteins are chains of amino acids that are essential to the production of antibodies, enzymes and hormones, and for maintaining normal pH levels in the body. They are necessary for proper growth of muscles, tendons, ligaments, hair and nails, repairing tissues and help provide energy for the body. There are two types of proteins depending upon the amino acid they supply: *complete and incomplete* proteins. Containing all the essential amino acids, complete proteins are found in foods like chicken, dairy, fish, meat, turkey and eggs. Lacking certain essential amino acids, incomplete proteins include beans, nuts/seeds, rice, peas, vegetables and whole grains. However, when two incomplete proteins are combined such as brown rice and beans, they form a complete protein. Whey protein is the highest quality and most complete protein because it contains all essential and non-essential amino acids. Eggs are another excellent source of protein that also contains vitamin D and other essential nutrients. Consuming a liquid protein such as milk after a workout helps to instantly nourish the muscles so they can begin to heal. Although body builders require additional protein, excessive protein intake may cause kidney and/or liver damage and can decrease the breakdown of fat for energy. The *biological value* (BV) of protein determines protein quality and is measured by how well amino acids are absorbed and utilized in the body. The following table is a list of biological values of common protein sources.

Biological Value (BV) of Protein Sources

Protein Sources	Biological Value
Whey Concentrates	104 - 159
Whey	100 - 104
Eggs	90 - 100
Egg Whites	85 - 90
Dairy (cottage cheese, milk, yogurt)	85 - 90
Chicken/Turkey	78 - 80
Fish	75 - 80
Beef	70 - 75
Soybeans	70 - 75
Brown Rice	65 - 70
Whole Wheat	60 - 65
Corn	60 - 65
Beans	55 - 60

Water

Essential for all absorptive, circulatory and digestive functions of the human body, water is nature's drink of life that helps maintain proper body temperature, flushes out inorganic substances and is necessary for transporting nutrients to our cells. Distilled water is the purest form of water because its vaporization process separates impurities from steam, which is then cooled and condenses back into water. Since all minerals are removed during the distillation process, it is important to drink distilled water with added electrolytes as well as fresh lemon juice. This is a great way to cleanse the kidneys and leach out excessive, unusable ionic forms of minerals that can cause harm if left inside the body. Reverse Osmosis (RO) is a high-quality filtration system that also removes impurities from the water. Mineral and spring water also contain naturally occurring minerals and are great healthy water options.

Tap water might not be as safe as you think. The long list of chemicals, toxins and impurities being discovered are rather alarming. In addition to heavy metals such as arsenic, copper, lead, iron and radon, some tap water has recently been found to contain asbestos, hormones, herbicides, pesticides and even pharmaceutical drugs. It has also been found to contain biological contaminants such as bacteria, viruses and parasites. One specific parasite, called *cryptosporidium,* is becoming a major problem here in the United States and is potentially fatal for people with HIV/AIDS or any immune system deficiency. Chlorine has been added to public drinking water for many years to kill bacteria and parasites. However, excessive amounts of chlorine are extremely toxic and higher levels of chlorine are being discovered in tap water. The Environmental Protection Agency (EPA) is working to reduce levels of chlorine in our drinking water amid some industry opposition. Fluoride is another substance added to water supplies, and believe it or not was once considered a lethal poison. Many contend it helps strengthens bones and teeth, but excessive amounts of fluoride are associated with cancer, osteoporosis and pitted teeth. As recently as January 2011, the Department of Health and Human Services and EPA have proposed to lower the recommended level of fluoride in tap water.

Not all tap water is unhealthy; it really depends on where you live. Each city processes and decontaminates their water supplies differently by using various chemicals and filters. The EPA advocates that tap water have a pH of 6.5 – 8.5, which are rather wide parameters of what is acceptable. Boiling water for 5 minutes helps kill bacteria, parasites and other impurities out of tap water. However, it has a tendency to concentrate lead contained in the water, so after boiling it is recommended to refrigerate the water for a while before drinking. The Water Quality Association (www.wqa.org) addresses inquiries about water purity and methods of treatment. NSF International (www.nsf.org) offers information on recommended water contaminant levels and water-quality issues. The EPA offers a toll-free Safe Drinking Water Hotline (800-426-4791) for certified water testing.

~ Micronutrients ~

Vitamins

Vitamins are organic compounds from plant and animal sources that are essential to a myriad of physiological processes like normalizing metabolism, lowering cholesterol and promoting good vision. They are considered *micronutrients* because they are only needed by the body in small amounts but are vital to health. Taking a high-quality multivitamin may be an effective way to help safeguard the body from nutritional deficiencies and other health disorders. Choosing a natural food source for obtaining vitamins is ideal; however in this fast-paced world we live in it is sometimes necessary to supplement some of these nutrients from a non-food source. Vitamins work best when taken with food, and are not meant to replace food by any means. They come in a variety of forms such as capsules, lozenges, tablets, powders, tinctures and in liquid form. Additional benefits from obtaining proper vitamin intake include increased coordination and brain function, assisting digestive disorders, promoting heart health, enhancing the immune system and reducing stress. Vitamins are also powerful antioxidants that reduce the risk of cancer, protect against bacterial and viral infections and help eliminate intestinal parasites. They work together with minerals in a balanced synergy - their combination is far greater than their individual effects.

Minerals

Minerals are naturally occurring inorganic substances formed through years of geological processes that contain specific crystalline chemical compositions and physical properties. Every living creature needs minerals for proper growth and sustained health. They support the nervous system, help the formation of bones, promote healthy muscle tone and strengthen the cardiovascular system. Similar to vitamins, minerals use enzymes as catalysts to optimize body functions, produce energy and are essential for proper nutrient absorption. There is a necessary balance needed between minerals because too much of one mineral can inhibit the positive effects of another. Conversely, a lack of minerals may raise the body's pH level and create an acidic environment suitable for cancer and other health disorders, so it is imperative to maintain adequate nutritional intake. The first group of minerals, called bulk minerals or *macrominerals,* include calcium, magnesium, phosphorus, potassium and sodium and are needed in large amounts. The second group of minerals, called trace minerals or *microminerals,* are only needed in small amounts and include boron, chromium, copper, germanium, iodine, iron, manganese, molybdenum, selenium, silicon, sulfur, vanadium and zinc.

Vitamins	Food Sources	Health Benefits
Vitamin A	apricots, asparagus, bell peppers (orange & red), broccoli, cantaloupe, carrots, cod liver oil, kale, mangoes, papayas, prunes, spinach, squash, sweet potatoes, Swiss chard, tomatoes, watercress	boosts immune system, protects against lung cancer, supports healthy bones/hair/skin/nails/teeth, helps lower blood pressure & cholesterol, promotes good vision, speeds wound healing
Vitamin B1 (Thiamine)	asparagus, beans, brewer's yeast, broccoli, brown rice, chicken, corn, eggplant, eggs, flaxseed, garlic, kale, kelp, lentils, millet, mushrooms, nuts/seeds, oatmeal, potatoes, salmon, spinach, tomatoes, whole grains	aids digestive disorders, stimulates brain function, enhances circulation, increases metabolism, improves muscle tone & coordination, sustains healthy growth, helps alleviate stress
Vitamin B2 (Riboflavin)	almonds, asparagus, avocados, beans, brewer's yeast, eggs, kale, kelp, millet, mushrooms, nuts/seeds, prunes, rice bran, salmon, soy foods, spinach, tomatoes, watercress, wheat germ, wild rice, yogurt	aids digestive disorders, red blood cell formation, increases metabolism, supports nervous system health, improves cardiovascular health, necessary for healthy growth, helps alleviate stress
Vitamin B3 (Niacin)	asparagus, barley, beef, brewer's yeast, buckwheat, cantaloupe, chicken, dates, eggs, liver (beef), mushrooms, nuts/seeds, peas, potatoes, rice bran, salmon, tomatoes, turkey, wheat bran, wild rice	aids digestive disorders, antibody production, increases circulation & metabolism, helps lower blood pressure & cholesterol, cardiovascular & nervous system health, helps alleviate stress
Vitamin B5 (Pantothenic Acid)	avocados, bananas, beans, beef, brewer's yeast, brown rice, cauliflower, chicken, eggs, kale, legumes, liver, mushrooms, nuts/seeds, oatmeal, salmon, soy flour, tomatoes, turkey, wheat germ, yogurt	aids digestive disorders, protects against anemia, improves cardiovascular health, promotes cell growth, increases metabolism, supports nervous system health, helps alleviate stress
Vitamin B6 (Pyridoxine)	avocados, bananas, beans, brewer's yeast, brown rice, cabbage, cantaloupe, carrots, chicken, eggs, kale, liver, molasses, potatoes, prunes, raisins, salmon, spinach, turkey, walnuts, wheat germ	aids digestive disorders, red blood cell formation, stimulates brain function, DNA/RNA synthesis, increases metabolism, supports nervous system health, helps alleviate stress
Vitamin B7 (Biotin)	almonds, barely, beans, beef, brewer's yeast, brown rice, cauliflower, egg yolks, legumes, mushrooms, oatmeal, peanuts, pecans, rice bran, soy foods, sunflower seeds, Swiss chard, turkey, wheat germ	aids digestive disorders, supports healthy hair/skin/nails, helps maintain blood sugar levels, increases metabolism, supports nervous system health, improves cardiovascular health
Vitamin B9 (Folic Acid)	asparagus, barley, beans, bran, brewer's yeast, broccoli, brown rice, cabbage, chicken, citrus fruits, dates, figs, leafy green vegetables, liver, nuts/seeds, oatmeal, peas, soy flour, wheat germ	aids digestive disorders, red blood cell formation, stimulates brain function, promotes cell growth, protects against lung cancer, supports nervous system health, helps alleviate stress

Vitamins	Food Sources	Health Benefits
Vitamin B12 (Cyanocobalamin)	alfalfa, apricots, beef, brewer's yeast, cereals, cheese, cod, eggs, figs, halibut, herring, mackerel, organ meats, oysters, poultry, salmon, shrimp, sea vegetables, swordfish, trout, tuna, whey, yogurt	aids digestive disorders, antibody & red blood cell formation, protects against anemia, increases metabolism, helps maintain fertility, prevents nerve damage, helps alleviate stress
Choline	almonds, apples, bananas, barley, beans (green, kidney), cauliflower, chicken, corn, egg yolks, flaxseeds, mushrooms (shitake), oranges, peanuts, potatoes, salmon, soy foods, tomatoes, turkey, whole grains	improves brain function & memory, lowers blood pressure & cholesterol, reduces inflammation, insomnia relief, supports gallbladder & liver health, assists transmission of nerve impulses
Inositol	almonds, bananas, berries, cabbage, cantaloupe, eggplant, grapefruit, lemons/limes, liver, milk, molasses, nuts, oats, oranges, organ meats, peas, raisins, sweet potatoes, tomatoes, whole grains	promotes calming effects, protects against diabetes & osteoporosis, supports liver health, lowers blood pressure & cholesterol, assists transmission of nerve impulses, stimulates brain function
Vitamin C	acerola, asparagus, bell peppers, berries, broccoli, cabbage (red), cantaloupe, guava, kale, kiwi, mangoes, onions, oranges, papayas, pineapple, spinach, strawberries, sweet potatoes, tomatoes	alleviates arthritis & inflammation, boosts immune system, improves cardiovascular health, reduces risk of cancer, lowers blood pressure & cholesterol, powerful antioxidant, improves healing
Vitamin D	alfalfa, cod liver oil, dairy, dandelion greens, egg yolks, halibut, herring, mackerel, mushrooms (shitake), oatmeal, roe, salmon, sardines, shrimp, soy foods, sweet potatoes, Swiss cheese, tuna	alleviates arthritis, normalizes blood clotting, improves calcium absorption, protects against skin cancer, reduces risk of diabetes, boosts immune system, healthy bones & teeth
Vitamin E	almonds, apricots (dried), asparagus, avocados, bell peppers, blueberries, cabbage, flaxseed, olives, papayas, pine nuts, prunes, salmon, spinach, tomatoes, watercress, wheat germ	alleviates arthritis, gout & inflammation, improves circulation, protects against Alzheimer's, reduces risk of cancer, improves muscle & nerve function, promotes eye, lung & prostate health
Vitamin K	alfalfa sprouts, asparagus, broccoli, Brussels sprouts, cabbage, cauliflower, cilantro, green tea, kale, molasses, olive & safflower oil, prunes, scallions, spinach, Swiss chard, watercress, whole wheat	normalizes blood clotting, protects against cancer & diabetes, increases calcium absorption, improves liver health, lowers blood pressure & cholesterol, protects against osteoporosis, eases menstrual pain

Minerals	Food Sources	Health Benefits
Boron	apples, apricots (dried), avocados, bananas, beans, cashews, carrots, grapes (red), hazelnuts, leafy green vegetables, oranges, peaches, peanuts, pears, raisins, tomatoes, walnuts, whole grains	improves alertness, stimulates brain function, helps increase testosterone levels, promotes muscle growth, increases metabolism, protects against osteoporosis
Calcium	almonds, artichokes, asparagus, broccoli, buckwheat, figs, herring, kelp, leafy green vegetables, milk, molasses, nuts/seeds, oats, raisins, salmon, soy foods, spinach, wheat bran, yogurt	assists blood clotting, normalizes heart rhythm, supports muscle function, promotes healthy hair, teeth & gums, protects against osteoporosis, helps prevent obesity, reduces muscle cramps
Chromium	apples, bananas, beef, bell peppers, brewer's yeast, broccoli, cabbage, carrots, chicken, eggs, garlic, grapes (red), mushrooms, onions, potatoes, spinach, tomatoes, turkey, wheat germ	protects DNA/RNA, regulates hunger, increases metabolism, helps control blood pressure & cholesterol, promotes pancreas & heart health, helps stabilize blood sugar
Cobalt	alfalfa, apricots, beef, broccoli, brewer's yeast, chicken, clams, eggs, figs, halibut, leafy green vegetables, milk, oats, salmon, sardines, shrimp, sea vegetables, spinach	protects against anemia, activates enzymes, reduces fatigue, promotes iron absorption, essential for red blood cell formation, increases nutrient absorption, supports nervous system health
Copper	asparagus, avocados, barley, beans, broccoli, buckwheat, eggplant, millet, molasses, mushrooms, nuts/seeds, oats (raw), olive oil, peas, radishes, raisins, spinach, squash, Swiss chard, tomatoes	protects against anemia, red blood cell formation, supports healthy bones & connective tissue, essential for enzymes & iron utilization, promotes eye/hair/skin health
Germanium	aloe vera juice, arugula, bran, carrots, celery, garlic, ginseng, kale, leafy green vegetables, mushrooms (shitake), onions, oysters, potatoes, sauerkraut, seeds, spinach, tomatoes, tuna	alleviates arthritis, boosts immune system, combats AIDS & cancer, increases cell oxygenation, stimulates circulation, protects against radiation damage, reduces risk of osteoporosis
Iodine	asparagus, cheese (cheddar, cottage, mozzarella), cod, eggs, garlic, haddock, kelp, lima beans, mushrooms, naan bread, salmon, sea salt, shellfish, soybeans, spinach, Swiss chard	stimulates brain function, necessary for normal growth & development, assists metabolism & thyroid function, reduces fatigue, helps eliminate toxins, supports healthy hair, skin, nails & teeth
Iron	almonds, avocados, beans, beef, beets, brewer's yeast, chicken, clams, eggs, figs, leafy green vegetables, liver, molasses, prunes, pumpkin seeds, raisins, sweet potatoes, wheat germ	protects against anemia, assists hemoglobin formation, healthy hair, skin & nails, boosts immune system, supplies oxygen to the body, regulates metabolism & body temperature
Magnesium	apricots, artichokes, avocados, bananas, beans, beets, brewer's yeast, brown rice, figs, kelp, kelp, millet, molasses, nuts/seeds, potatoes, raisins, salmon, soy foods, spinach, whole grains	alleviates asthma & migraines, helps lower blood pressure & cholesterol, protects against diabetes & osteoporosis, increases calcium absorption, supports kidney health

Minerals	Food Sources	Health Benefits
Manganese	alfalfa, bananas, barley, blueberries, bran, brown rice, Brussels sprouts, celery, egg yolks, garlic, legumes, millet, nuts, oats, pineapple, raisins, spinach, sweet potatoes	supports healthy bones/cartilage, helps control blood sugar, protects against osteoporosis, improves digestion, boosts immune system, eases PMS symptoms
Molybdenum	apricots, broccoli, brown rice, buckwheat, cabbage, cantaloupe, cauliflower, eggs, molasses, onions, peas, potatoes, spinach, sunflower seeds, wheat germ	protects against anemia, lowers risk of impotence, reduces risk of esophageal cancer, supports enzyme function, strengthens bones/teeth, liver detoxifier
Phosphorus	almonds, asparagus, beef, bran, brewer's yeast, chicken, corn, dairy, eggs, garlic, halibut, lentils,peanuts, pumpkin seeds, salmon, turkey, whole grains, yogurt	aids digestion, necessary for blood clotting, promotes proper brain function & heart rhythm, helps balance hormones, essential for bones/teeth, promotes cell growth
Potassium	apples, apricots, avocados, bananas, brewer's yeast, brown rice, cantaloupe, figs, molasses, oranges, raisins, spinach, sunflower seeds, tomatoes, whole grains	promotes heart/kidney/nervous system health, maintains muscle function, insomnia relief, regulates blood pressure, improves brain/lung function, eases stress
Selenium	alfalfa, barley, beef, Brazil nuts, brewer's yeast, broccoli, brown rice, chicken, eggs, kelp, liver, molasses, onions, salmon, Swiss chard, tuna, turkey, wheat germ	alleviates arthritis & asthma, protects against cancer, boosts immune system, supports male fertility, lowers blood pressure & cholesterol
Silicon	alfalfa, almonds, apples, beets, bell peppers, brown rice, cabbage, celery, cherries, eggplant, leafy green vegetables, pumpkin, raisins, soybeans, whole grains	aids calcium absorption, combats Alzheimer's disease by reducing aluminum absorption, boosts immune system, promotes healthy bones/skin/teeth
Sodium	almost all foods contain some sodium	alleviates cramps & headaches, helps maintain proper pH levels, essential for proper brain, enzyme, muscle & nerve function, helps relieve depression
Sulfur	artichokes, asparagus, beans, broccoli, Brussels sprouts, cabbage, eggs, flaxseeds, garlic, kale, onions, radishes, sauerkraut, spinach, whole grains, yogurt	improves blood circulation, protects against diverticulitis, hypoglycemia & osteoporosis, promotes skin integrity, boosts immune system
Vanadium	apples, beets, buckwheat, cabbage, carrots, millet, mushrooms, sunflower seeds, onions, plums, radishes, tomatoes, vegetable oils (olive/safflower)	protects against diabetes, lowers risk of cardiovascular disease, supports cholesterol metabolism, helps lower blood pressure, promotes healthy bones/teeth
Zinc	beef, brewer's yeast, buckwheat, eggs, garlic, ginger, kelp, mushrooms, nuts/seeds, oysters, pumpkin seeds, salmon, sardines, soy foods, spinach	supports prostate health, helps alleviates acne, lowers blood pressure/cholesterol, boosts immune system, protects against diabetes, assists wound healing

~ Nutritional Deficiencies ~

Nutritional deficiencies are linked to an increased risk of many degenerative health disorders. Listed below are vitamins and minerals with common symptoms that are associated with each deficiency.

Vitamin Deficiencies & Associated Disorders

Vitamin A – acne, allergies, anemia, boils, cold sores, color & night blindness, dry hair & skin, eye infections, fatigue, growth impairment, increased risk of skin cancer, insomnia, jaundice, kidney stones, loss of appetite, loss of smell, macular degeneration, moles, painful joints, peeling nails, reproductive & respiratory disorders, warts, weakened immune system, weight loss, wrinkles

Vitamin B1 (Thiamine) – confusion, constipation, difficulty breathing, digestive disorders, edema, fatigue, gangrene, irritability, loss of appetite, memory loss, muscle atrophy, numbness, Raynaud's disease, sore muscles, weakness, weight loss

Vitamin B2 (Riboflavin) – acne, blurred vision, cataracts, cognitive impairment, cracked lips, dandruff, dermatitis, dizziness, eczema, inflammation/sores on tongue, insomnia, itchy/burning eyes, macular degeneration, oily hair, poor digestion, sensitivity to light, skin lesions, vaginal itching

Vitamin B3 (Niacin) – canker sores, dementia, depression, dermatitis, diarrhea, fatigue, halitosis, headaches, impaired digestion, insomnia, loss of appetite, low blood sugar, nausea, sore tongue, weakness

Vitamin B5 (Pantothenic Acid) – abdominal pain, Addison's disease, allergies, anxiety, depression, eczema, fatigue, gout, graying hair, hair loss, headaches, indigestion, insomnia, muscle spasms, nausea, numbness, physiological disorders, poor coordination

Vitamin B6 (Pyridoxine) – acne, Addison's disease, anemia, arthritis, boils, blurred vision, canker sores, carpal tunnel syndrome, celiac disease, cold sores, depression, eczema, fatigue, hair loss, halitosis, headaches, impaired hearing, irritability, loss of appetite, macular degeneration, memory loss, migraines, nausea, numbness, rashes, Raynaud's disease, sensitivity to sunlight, sore tongue, slow-healing wounds

Vitamin B7 (Biotin) – anemia, depression, dermatitis, hair loss, high blood sugar, insomnia, loss of appetite, muscle pain/weakness, nausea, pale skin, sore tongue

Vitamin B9 (Folic Acid) – anemia, anxiety, birth defects, depression, difficulty breathing, digestive disorders, fatigue, graying hair, insomnia, memory loss, pale skin, slow metabolism, weakness

Vitamin B12 (Cyanocobalamin) – Alzheimer's disease, anemia, anxiety, bone loss, difficulty breathing, constipation, depression, digestive disorders, fatigue, glaucoma, headaches, irregular heartbeat, insomnia, malabsorption, memory loss, migraines, neurological problems, restlessness, shingles, sore tongue, spinal cord deterioration

Choline – arteriosclerosis, cardiovascular decline, digestive disorders, epilepsy, fatigue, fatty liver, folate deficiency, high blood pressure, impaired fetal development, increased triglyceride levels,

insomnia, kidney & liver disorders, Parkinson's disease, ulcers
Inositol – anxiety, arteriosclerosis, constipation, hair loss, increased cholesterol levels, irritability, skin disorders

Vitamin C – acne, Addison's disease, anemia, bleeding gums, boils, bruising, cataracts, cold sores, depression, digestive disorders, eczema, fatigue, gingivitis, glaucoma, irritability, jaundice, loose teeth, moles, nose bleeds, rashes, scurvy, shingles, slow-healing wounds, stress, warts, weakened immune system, wrinkles

Vitamin D – brittle bones, decreased calcium absorption, diarrhea, fatigue, insomnia, irregular heartbeat, irritability, kidney & liver disorders, loss of appetite, osteoporosis, pale skin, rickets, sensitivity to pain, slow metabolism, thyroid disorders, visual problems, weight loss

Vitamin E – anemia, bed sores, cardiovascular decline, cataracts, decreased circulation, dry hair, enlarged prostate, gangrene, gastrointestinal disorders, hair loss, impaired reflexes and muscle coordination, impaired speech and/or vision, impotence, infertility, jaundice, leg cramps, menstrual problems, miscarriages, moles, premature birth, red blood cell damage, shingles, warts, weakness

Vitamin K – brittle bones, excessive bleeding, high blood sugar, low platelet count

Mineral Deficiencies & Associated Disorders

Boron (*rare*) – acne, anemia, arthritis, cognitive impairment, eczema, inflammation, memory loss, reduced mineral absorption, osteoporosis

Calcium – anxiety, arthritis, birth defects, brittle bones, cardiovascular decline, cognitive impairment, convulsions, cramps, depression, eczema, high blood pressure & cholesterol, Insomnia, irregular bone growth, muscle spasms, osteoporosis, rickets, tooth decay

Chromium – anxiety, arteriosclerosis, diabetes, fatigue, glucose intolerance, high cholesterol & triglyceride levels, poor digestion, weight loss

Cobalt – anemia, anorexia, malabsorption, nervous system disorders, vitamin B12 deficiency

Copper – anemia, depression, diarrhea, fatigue, fragile bones, hair loss, hyperthyroidism, respiratory decline, skin lesions, weakness

Germanium (*rare*) – no established levels of deficiency to date, however a lack of germanium has been associated with arthritis, asthma, cardiovascular impairment, high blood pressure, increased risk of cancer & viral infections, osteoporosis, weakened immune system

Iodine – fatigue, hypothyroidism, increased risk of breast cancer, mental retardation, weight gain

Iron – anemia, anxiety, brittle nails, cognitive impairment, constipation, depression, difficulty swallowing, dizziness, dry hair, fatigue, hair loss, inflamed tongue, mouth lesions

Magnesium – anxiety, asthma, cardiovascular decline, confusion, depression, fatigue, high blood pressure, insomnia, irregular heartbeat, irritable bowel syndrome, kidney stones, migraines, poor digestion, respiratory decline, seizures, weakness

Manganese (*rare*) – atherosclerosis, convulsions, ear & eye disorders, excessive sweating, fatigue, glucose intolerance, hearing loss, high blood pressure & cholesterol, increased heart rate, irritability, memory loss, muscle cramps, ringing in ears, tooth grinding

Molybdenum – gum & mouth disorders, impotence, increased risk of cancer

Phosphorus (*rare*) – anxiety, anorexia, bone & skin sensitivity, cognitive impairment, difficulty breathing, fatigue, irritability, joint stiffness, loss of appetite, numbness, poor bone development, weakness, weight loss

Potassium – acne, chills, cognitive impairment, constipation, depression, diarrhea, edema, excessive thirst, glucose intolerance, high cholesterol, impaired growth, irregular heartbeat, insomnia, irritability, low blood pressure, muscle fatigue, nausea, respiratory decline, salt retention, slower reflexes

Selenium – fatigue, high cholesterol, hyperthyroidism, impaired growth, increased risk of cancer & cardiovascular disease, inflammation, liver disorders, muscle pain, pancreas malfunction, sterility, weakened red blood cells

Silicon – brittle nails, cardiovascular decline, dry/frizzy/thin hair, hair loss, hormonal changes, increased risk of Alzheimer's disease & senility, irregular bone growth, osteoporosis, premature aging, sensitivity to cold, weakened immune system, wrinkles

Sodium (*rare*) – abdominal cramps, anorexia, confusion, dehydration, depression, fatigue, flatulence, frequent infections, headaches, irregular heartbeat, loss of coordination, low blood pressure, muscle cramps, nausea, poor memory, seizures, weakness, weight loss

Sulfur – acne, arthritis, asthma, circulatory disorders, constipation, dry skin, inflammation, migraines, muscle pain, stress, urinary tract disorders, weakened immune system, wrinkles

Vanadium – cardiovascular decline, high cholesterol & triglyceride levels, kidney disorders, reproductive impairment

Zinc – acne, brittle nails, diabetes, diarrhea, depression, eczema, fatigue, growth impairment, hair loss, high cholesterol, impotence/infertility, loss of appetite, loss of smell and taste, low birth weight, memory loss, mental retardation, peeling nails, poor night vision, prostate disorders, skin lesions, slow-healing wounds, wcakcncd immunc systcm

Part Two

Super Foods, Natural Supplements, Therapeutic Spices & Holistic Herbs

~ Super Foods ~

Almonds – (vitamins B2 & E, copper, magnesium, manganese, phosphorous, potassium, tryptophan)
Cultivated throughout the Mediterranean and in California, raw almonds are a nutritious, high quality protein rich in antioxidants, omega-3 fatty acids and phytonutrients that help lower cholesterol levels, protect against cell damage and reduce the risk of cancer. They are rich in monounsaturated fats like olive oil and have been linked to lowering the risk of atherosclerosis, cardiovascular disease, digestive disorders, gallstones, high blood pressure and diabetes. Almonds protect against osteoporosis by helping to increase bone density, and are rich in copper and iron which is beneficial for those who are anemic. Almonds contain vitamin E, and food sources rich in this anti-aging vitamin are associated with strengthening the heart muscle, improving circulation and reducing the risk of Alzheimer's disease. Additionally, almonds are an excellent source of highly absorbable protein that helps muscles recover faster from a hard workout, increases natural energy production and helps stimulates weight loss.

Apples – (vitamin C, dietary fiber)
With more than 10,000 varieties grown around the world, apples are a delicious, mouth-watering fruit rich in vitamin C and dietary fiber. Revered by the ancient Greeks and Romans, they contain powerful phytonutrients that help protect the body from harmful environmental toxins, inhibit the proliferation of tumors, and have been effective for lowering blood pressure and cholesterol levels. Apples are a great source of boron, a trace mineral that increases mental alertness by affecting electrical activity in the brain. For people who smoke, apples are your new best friend! They are rich in pectin which improves lung function and reduces the risk of lung cancer. Pectin actually binds to carcinogens, heavy metals, environmental toxins and nitrates from cured meats, and eliminates them from the body before they can be absorbed. Apples are linked to reducing the risk of asthma and bronchitis, and are rich in dietary fiber so they are beneficial for diabetics. They also help increase bone strength, improve bowel function and stimulate weight loss. Furthermore, apples include anti-aging properties that help prevent wrinkles, and for postmenopausal women green apples may help raise estrogen levels.

Apricots – (vitamins A & C, potassium)
Originally cultivated in China, Persia and throughout the Mediterranean, apricots are flavorful summer fruits that are rich in life-extending nutrients that are known to be beneficial for numerous health disorders. They contain dietary fiber, lycopene and other powerful antioxidants that help neutralize

toxins, protect cells and strengthen tissues, lower blood pressure and cholesterol levels and promote heart health. Enjoyed by many ancient civilizations, apricots have been effective for inhibiting tumor growth, reducing the risk of peptic ulcers and easing digestive disorders such as indigestion, constipation and diverticulitis. These sweet fruits produce an alkaline reaction in the body which helps protect against premature aging, acidosis and heartburn. Mainly grown domestically in California, apricots are rich in beta carotene which reduces the risk of cataracts and macular degeneration, and through regular consumption may significantly reduce the risk of prostate cancer.

Artichokes – (vitamins A, B, C & K, calcium, folate, iron, magnesium, potassium)
Native to the Mediterranean and a member of the milk thistle family, artichokes have been used for centuries to help improve gallbladder, digestive and liver function. Respected and widely utilized by the Greeks and Romans, they are very low in saturated fats and provide many health benefits like cleansing the blood, lowering cholesterol and triglyceride levels, stabilizing blood sugar, and are safe to eat for both diabetics and those who have Celiac disease. Rich in wholesome nutrients, artichokes are known for improving conditions of cirrhosis and hepatitis by stimulating cell and tissue regeneration in the liver. They also contain *caffeoylquinic acids* which are natural compounds that may inhibit the ability of the HIV virus to reproduce. Additional benefits of this super food include alleviating symptoms of diarrhea, indigestion, irritable bowel syndrome and Crohn's disease, and enhancing skin luminosity by flushing out excess water and toxins from the body.

Avocados – (vitamins B6, C, E & K, copper, folate, potassium)
Native to Mexico, Central and South America, avocados contain monounsaturated fats (oleic acid), polyunsaturated fats (linoleic acid) and dietary fiber that help lower LDL (bad) cholesterol levels, increase HDL (good) cholesterol levels and protect against cardiovascular disease. Although their fat content is approximately 20%, more than most other fruits, avocados are still regarded as a heart-healthy food. Known in Jamaica as the "alligator pear" due to its skin texture, avocados are rich in phytonutrients that may help reduce the risk of breast, oral and prostate cancer. They have also been known to help regulate blood sugar levels, improve circulatory disorders, increase the absorption of beta carotene and are effective for eliminating free radicals from the body. The "Hass" avocado is the most popular grown in California, and even though they are at their best during the spring and summer months, they are the only variety of avocado that is able to grow year-round.

Bananas – (vitamins B6 & C, manganese, potassium)

Cultivated in Malaysia some 4,000 years ago, bananas are a sweet, tropical fruit that provide protein, dietary fiber, amino acids and organic sugars that are a great source of natural energy. They are rich in potassium - an electrolyte that helps regulate heart function, protects against osteoporosis, lowers blood pressure levels and helps lower the risk of cardiovascular disease. Also available as plantains, bananas contain numerous antioxidants that help lower the risk of cancer, kidney disease and increase the absorption of nutrients in the body. Bananas are also rich in pectin and soluble fiber which lowers cholesterol, alleviates constipation and diarrhea, is soothing to the digestive tract and helps protect against peptic ulcers. Additional benefits of these tasty cereal toppers include strengthening the immune system, improving eyesight and quieting a cough.

Barley – (vitamins A, B1, B3, B5 & K, folate, iron, magnesium, phosphorus, potassium, selenium)

Originating around 8000 B.C. in Mesopotamia, barley is one of the oldest cultivated crops and provides many healthful benefits. This nutty-flavored, nutritious whole grain contains oleic and linolenic fatty acids which are known for reducing the risk of arthritis and atherosclerosis, improving liver and muscle function and helping to lower blood pressure and cholesterol levels. Barley is beneficial for improving digestive health by feeding "friendly" bacteria to the intestinal tract to relieve gallstones, hemorrhoids and reduce the risk of colon cancer. The rich fiber content of barley also helps protect against diabetes, breast cancer, improves cardiovascular health and is beneficial for post-menopausal women. Once a staple cereal of ancient gladiators and formerly traded as currency, barely is now primarily used as a component of health food, as a malt base for beer and as animal feed for domesticated livestock.

Beans – (vitamins A, B1, B2, B3 C & K, folate, iron, magnesium, molybdenum, potassium)

Including black, garbanzo, green, lima, navy, pinto, red and soy, beans are rich in protein, water soluble vitamins and are loaded with antioxidants that help protect against cardiovascular disease. They have shown promise in protecting against many forms of cancer, contain powerful anti-aging properties and help lower blood pressure and cholesterol levels. Beans are also a rich source of dietary fiber which promotes regularity, cleans the digestive tract, and helps stabilize blood sugar levels by preventing them from rising too rapidly after meals. This is especially beneficial for people with diabetes, insulin resistance or hypoglycemia. When beans are mixed with whole grains such as brown rice or quinoa, they create an ideal, virtually fat-free, high-quality protein combination. Fava beans (broad beans) are high in dietary fiber and protein; however there are some nutritional concerns that should be addressed.

Some people unknowingly have an enzyme deficiency called *glucose-6-phosphate dehydrogenase* (G6PD) that, when fava beans are consumed, causes "favism" which is characterized by hemolytic anemia (breaking up of red blood cells). Fava beans are excessively rich in potassium and phosphorus which may lead to kidney problems or kidney failure. They should be avoided by those who take MAO inhibitors, and have a high glycemic index (GI) score so they should also be avoided by diabetics.

Beets – (vitamins A, B9 & C, calcium, iron, magnesium, manganese, phosphorous, potassium)
Native to the Mediterranean and North Africa, beets were originally cultivated by the ancient Romans and are one of the strongest anti-cancer foods available. The vital nutrients found in this crimson-colored vegetable are effective for cleansing the liver, and are important for pregnant women because they help reduce the risk of spina bifida and other neural tube defects. The combination of beet fiber and *betacyanin*, the ruby-red pigment giving beets their color, helps lower the risk of colon and stomach cancer and increases white blood cell count. Beets are also known for improving cardiovascular health, alleviating arthritis and inflammation and are beneficial for those with anemia by naturally manufacturing red blood cells. Additionally, they help stimulate the lymph glands, protect against arteriosclerosis and atherosclerosis, and are rich in calcium which promotes strong bones and reduces the risk of osteoporosis.

Bell Peppers – (vitamins A, B1, B6, B9, C, E, K, folate, manganese, potassium)
Coming in a variety of vivid colors like red, orange, yellow, green and purple, bell peppers are excellent for preventative health because they contain folate and powerful antioxidants that alleviate arthritis, neutralize toxins and help prevent premature aging. Native to South America, these crisp, fresh-tasting veggies are rich in vitamin C and dietary fiber, and are known for reducing the risk of bladder, cervix, colon, lung, pancreas and prostate cancer as well as lowering cholesterol levels. They are effective for promoting weight loss, and help alleviate respiratory disorders such as asthma and bronchitis. Bell peppers contain nutrients like *capsaicin* and *flavonoids* that help prevent blood clots, reduce the risk of atherosclerosis, and improve lung function. Red bell peppers also contain the antioxidant *lycopene* that promotes healthy vision by protecting against disorders like cataracts and macular degeneration.

Berries – (vitamins C & E, iron, manganese, potassium)
Including blackberries, blueberries, boysenberries, cherries, cranberries, raspberries and strawberries, this tasty bunch contains a synergy of powerful antioxidants that significantly reduce the risk of cancer,

improve cardiovascular health and are beneficial for degenerative eye disorders like cataracts and macular degeneration. Antioxidants are effective for protecting the brain from oxidative stress, slowing down the process of premature aging by promoting healthy skin, and may help reduce the risk of senility and Alzheimer's disease. In smoothies or just as they are, berries are rich in phytonutrients that help lower blood pressure and cholesterol levels, inhibit the growth of tumors and help stabilize blood sugar levels. Cherries provide important nutrients like potassium, vitamins A and C, and have a low glycemic index (GI) score. But they are high in sodium, and are not recommended for low-sodium diets or for those who have high blood pressure.

Broccoli – (vitamins A, B1, B2, B3, B5, B6, C, E & K, chromium, folate, iron, zinc)
Related to the cabbage family and native to Europe, broccoli is an excellent source of beta-carotene, calcium and fiber, and is one of the strongest anti-cancer and antiviral foods that nature provides. This heart-smart vegetable contains powerful antioxidants that help reduce the risk of breast, colon, cervical and many other forms of cancer. The phytonutrients in broccoli assist in destroying leukemia and melanoma cells, inhibit the growth of tumors and ulcers and help protect against birth defects. Rich in dietary fiber, they help regulate insulin and blood sugar levels, lower blood pressure and cholesterol levels, promote cardiovascular health and relieve digestive disorders such as indigestion and constipation. Tasty whether raw or cooked, broccoli also strengthens the immune system, helps stimulate weight loss, protects against osteoporosis by increasing bone strength, and contains lutein which is known to protect against vision disorders.

Brown Rice – (vitamin B, magnesium, manganese, selenium, tryptophan)
Native to Asia and Africa, rice is a staple food for millions of people and is the most consumed food in the world. Brown rice is an excellent source of essential fatty acids and is effective for lowering blood pressure and cholesterol levels and protecting against cardiovascular disease. Its mineral content produces energy from protein and carbohydrates which are important for maintaining a healthy nervous system. Brown rice is rich in fiber which helps protect against coronary heart disease and colon cancer, stimulates weight loss, and eases digestive disorders like constipation and irritable bowel syndrome. Even though it is beneficial for stabilizing blood sugar levels, brown rice has a medium glycemic index (GI) score and should be consumed in moderation by those are diabetic. Brown rice is a "gluten-free" grain and is safe to eat for those who have Celiac disease. Other healthy rice alternatives are basmati and long-grain rice, which have a lower glycemic index score than jasmine, short-grain or white rice.

Buckwheat – (fiber, iron, magnesium, manganese, tryptophan)

Native to Asia and widely cultivated in China around the 10th century, buckwheat has been utilized for centuries as an energizing and nutritious component to a healthy diet. This gluten-free grain is rich in dietary fiber and powerful phytonutrients that help alleviate asthma, control blood sugar levels, lower blood pressure and cholesterol and improve cardiovascular health. Buckwheat is actually harvested as a fruit seed and contains plant lignans that help protect against benign prostatic hypertrophy (BPH) as well as breast cancer, colon and prostate cancer. The flavonoids *rutin* and *quercitin* found in buckwheat increase the antioxidant power of vitamin C, and are effective for preventing blood clots and maintaining proper blood flow. Additional benefits include alleviating gallstones, easing irritable bowel syndrome and improving intestinal flora. Even though buckwheat is gluten-free, it is often processed and cross-contaminated with other gluten grains. **For those who have celiac disease, it is extremely important to read nutrition labels for buckwheat flour that is processed in a "gluten-free" environment.*

Cabbage – (vitamins A, B1, B2, B6, C, E & K, calcium, folate, magnesium, manganese, potassium)

Originating in Asia and loaded with antioxidants, cabbage is a low-calorie, nutrient-dense food that is known as the "king" of cruciferous vegetables. It contains antibacterial and antiviral properties, and organic substances called *indole glucosinolates* that help lower the risk of breast, colon, ovarian and stomach cancer. The nutrients in cabbage also improve cardiovascular health, help protect against lung cancer and may reduce a smoker's risk by more than 60%. Men living in Asia and parts of Europe experience much lower rates of prostate cancer than Americans partly due to consuming more vegetable-rich diets containing this staple food. Furthermore, cabbage is also effective for improving skin infections, wounds, ulcers and tumors, and contains high levels of iron and sulfur that assist in cleaning the digestive system and improving gastrointestinal health. Both green and red cabbages are rich in vitamins and minerals, reduce the toxic effects of alcohol on the liver and may help protect brain cells against the onset of Alzheimer's disease.

Cantaloupe – (vitamins A, B3, B6 & C, dietary fiber, folate, potassium)

Native to Africa, Asia and Persia, cantaloupes are a sweet summer melon loaded with beta carotene and vitamin C that help reduce the risk of cardiovascular disease, emphysema and lung cancer. Named after the papal gardens of Cantaloupe, Italy, and enjoyed for centuries by ancient Greek and Roman civilizations, the health benefits of cantaloupes are extensive as they help strengthen the immune system, increase energy production, stimulate metabolism, stabilize blood sugar levels and neutralize harmful toxins. This refreshing fruit is also helps lower blood pressure and cholesterol, improves respiratory health and reduces the risk of developing cataracts and macular degeneration. Additionally, cantaloupes have an alkalizing effect on the body which helps protect against premature aging, acidosis, cancer, heartburn, indigestion and numerous other degenerative disorders.

Carrots – (vitamins A, B, C & K, magnesium, potassium)
Originally cultivated in Asia and the Middle East, carrots are the richest vegetable source of beta carotene and are loaded with many other powerful antioxidants that help protect against lung cancer, cardiovascular disease, cataracts and macular degeneration. These sweet snacks are associated with reducing the risk of postmenopausal breast cancer, and cancers of the bladder, cervix, larynx, esophagus and prostate. Carrots contain a phytonutrient called *falcarinol* that is linked to lowering the risk of colon cancer as well. Furthermore, the abundance of beta carotene in carrots helps reduce the risk of heart attack and stroke, strengthens the immune system, protects cells against toxins and is beneficial for alleviating asthma and bronchitis.

Cauliflower – (vitamins B1, B2, B3, B5, B6, C & K, folate, magnesium, potassium)
Native to Asia and an excellent source of protein and vitamin C, cauliflower is a potent anti-cancer food that is beneficial for detoxifying the liver and eliminating carcinogens from the body. This cruciferous vegetable is rich in dietary fiber and powerful phytonutrients that help lower blood pressure and cholesterol, protect against cirrhosis and hepatitis, improve kidney health and help alleviate cystic fibrosis. Cauliflower produces a sulfur compound when consumed that inhibits some tumors from proliferating, and may help reduce the risk of many forms of cancer such as bladder, breast, colon, lung, ovarian and prostate. It is also beneficial for supporting bladder health, as well as improving numerous digestive disorders such as constipation, colitis, Crohn's disease and irritable bowel syndrome. Additional health benefits include improving cardiovascular function, reducing inflammation, lowering the risk of Type 2 diabetes and protecting against obesity.

Celery – (vitamins A, B1, B2, B6, C & K, calcium, folate, iron, magnesium, phosphorus, potassium)
Celery is a crunchy, slightly salty, heart-healthy vegetable that is widely used across various cultures and cuisines. Before it was used as a food, celery was known to the ancient Greeks for its ability to lower blood pressure and cholesterol, reduce arthritis and inflammation, improve cardiovascular health and correct urinary tract disorders. Brewed as a drink, celery was also popular in the Orient for

improving digestive disorders like constipation, indigestion and irritable bowel syndrome. It is an excellent source of vitamin K which promotes healthy blood clotting, protects against atherosclerosis, controls blood-sugar levels for diabetics and helps alleviate menstrual pain. Celery enables the body to better absorb calcium which increases bone strength and reduces the risk of osteoporosis. This super food inhibits the growth of tumors and ulcers, and helps protect against many forms of cancer such as bladder, breast, colon, lung, ovarian, pancreatic, prostate, stomach and testicular. Celery has also been effective for cystic fibrosis and hepatitis, as well as respiratory disorders like asthma and bronchitis.

Figs – (vitamins A, B1, B2, calcium, iron, manganese, potassium)
Originally cultivated in Egypt, figs are excellent sources of dietary fiber that help normalize constipation and indigestion, and protect against obesity by stimulating metabolism. This nutritious fruit contains trace minerals like iron and potassium that increase energy levels, help lower blood pressure and cholesterol and improve cardiovascular function. Figs are rich in antioxidants that reduce the risk of colon and breast cancer, promote liver health and help normalize the body's pH. They contain anti-diabetic properties which helps maintain normal blood sugar levels, and may lower the amount of insulin injections needed by diabetes patients. Figs also protect against osteoporosis by increasing bone density, and help reduce the amount of calcium lost as we age by counteracting high-sodium diets. Additional benefits include easing respiratory disorders like asthma, bronchitis and whooping cough, and protecting against vision disorders such as cataracts and macular degeneration.

Grapefruit – (vitamins A, B5 & C, folate, potassium)
Native to the West Indies and considered to be one of the "Seven Wonders of Barbados," grapefruits are rich in vitamin C and dietary fiber. This tart and tangy citrus fruit helps strengthen the immune system, protects against the common cold, neutralizes toxins and contains anti-inflammatory properties that help alleviate asthma and bronchitis. Grapefruits contain powerful phytonutrients that lower the risk of cardiovascular disease, inhibit tumor growth and reduce the risk of breast, colon, lung, prostate and stomach cancer. Along with grapefruit juice, they are also beneficial for protecting against atherosclerosis, lowering blood pressure and cholesterol, normalizing pH levels, eliminating kidney stones and improving liver function by increasing enzyme production. Grapefruit seed extract, not be confused with grape seed extract, is simply the liquid derived from the pulp and seeds of the grapefruit and is also available as a health food supplement. It provides beneficial alkalizing effects for the body, and contains powerful antibiotic properties that protect against bacteria, viruses and intestinal parasites.

__Grapes__ (*red*) – (__vitamins B1, B6 & C, manganese, potassium__)

Enjoyed by ancient Greek and Roman civilizations, red grapes are a tasty summer snack, a great source of antioxidants and contain potent phytonutrients called *flavonoids* which give them their reddish-purple color. These healthful nutrients are effective against vascular disorders by slowing the formation of blood clots, protecting against varicose veins, reducing cholesterol damage to the arteries and have shown the ability to reverse atherosclerosis. Red grapes are also known to lower the risk of breast, colon, lung and prostate cancer, and protect against cardiovascular disease. They are also beneficial for stimulating metabolism, improving lung function and contain anti-inflammatory properties that help alleviate asthma and bronchitis. Another phytonutrient found in red grapes and red wine called *resveratrol,* a powerful antioxidant that helps slow the aging process, and is linked to reducing the build up of plaque in the brain associated with Alzheimer's disease.

__Green Tea__ (*decaf*) – (__vitamins B1, B2, B3, B5 & C, potassium, zinc__)

Originally cultivated in China, green tea contains many powerful antioxidants and other nutritional compounds that help protect against most forms of cancer. The catechin *epigallocatechin gallate* (EGCG) found in green tea is able to penetrate the body's cells and protect DNA against environmental toxins. Green tea is beneficial for regulating blood sugar levels, lowering blood pressure and cholesterol levels, supporting the immune system and stimulating weight loss. Providing antibacterial and antiviral properties, it is also effective for alleviating mental fatigue, improving tooth decay and may slow the onset of atherosclerosis. For men, drinking green tea daily is extremely important for reducing the risk of esophageal, laryngeal, lung and prostate cancer. EGCG may even help reduce amyloid plaques from forming around the brain associated with dementia and Alzheimer's disease.

__Honey__ (*raw*) – (__vitamins B2 & B6, iron, manganese__)

An organic alternative to white sugar, raw honey contains antibacterial, antifungal and antiviral properties that inhibit tumor production and help lower the risk of cancer. Made naturally by bees, this savory sweetener contains friendly bacteria called *lactobacillus* responsible for its therapeutic properties. Raw honey has been effective for alleviating upper respiratory infections, stimulating the immune system, lowering cholesterol and easing allergies. It is also known for increasing energy and athletic performance, and assisting muscle repair for athletes and weightlifters. When used topically, raw honey is an effective antiseptic for improving skin ailments such as burns, wounds and ulcers. Natural, unprocessed honey provides more nutrients and causes a much lower rise in blood sugar than refined or table sugars do. When it is heated and processed, most of the valuable phytonutrients are eliminated. Since honey has a wide glycemic index (GI) range, diabetics should consume in moderation only.

Kale – (vitamins A, B1, B2, B3, C, E & K, calcium, folate, iron, magnesium, manganese, potassium)
Kale is a leafy green vegetable that is part of the cruciferous family, and provides more nutrition for fewer calories than most other foods. It contains sulfur-based phytonutrients that help protect against breast, colon, lung, ovarian, prostate and stomach cancer even if genetically susceptible. Kale reduces the risk of cardiovascular disease, helps lower blood pressure and cholesterol and detoxifies the body. It has been effective for alleviating arthritis and inflammation, strengthening the immune system and may help slow mental decline. This super-green food is also beneficial for those who have hyperthyroidism because it suppresses thyroid function. Kale is a great source of dietary fiber that improves digestive disorders such as constipation, IBS and indigestion, and is rich in calcium which protects against osteoporosis. It also helps normalize pH levels, and contains powerful *carotenoids* that reduce the risk of cataracts, macular degeneration and other eye-related disorders.

Kelp (*sea vegetables*) – (vitamin K, calcium, folate, iodine, iron, magnesium, tryptophan)
One of the most nutritious foods on the planet, sea vegetables contain powerful anti-cancer properties and nearly all minerals found in the human body. The phytonutrients in kelp have shown to inhibit tumor growth, alleviate asthma and bronchitis and help remove heavy metals from the body. They are also beneficial for correcting digestive disorders and obesity associated with menopause, and reducing the risk of postmenopausal breast cancer. Rich in iodine and folate, sea vegetables increase thyroid function and are beneficial for those who have an underactive thyroid, or hypothyroidism. Iodine is known to help regulate metabolism and promote healthy brain development; conversely a deficiency of iodine is linked to mental retardation in children and may lead to compromised intelligence and lowered mental abilities. Folate deficiencies have been associated with atherosclerosis, colon cancer, heart attack and stroke. Other nutritious sea vegetables include agar, arame, dulse, hijiki, kombu, nori & wakame.

Lemons/Limes – (vitamin C)
Originally cultivated in Asia and India, both lemons and limes are excellent sources of vitamin C and contain powerful antioxidant and antibiotic properties. Vitamin C neutralizes free radicals that damage cell membranes, and contain powerful phytonutrients called *flavonoids* that inhibit the growth of cancer cells. Naturally tart and sour, these citrus fruits protect against bladder, lung and skin cancer, help

stimulate the immune system and are associated with lowering the risk of cardiovascular disease. Lemons and limes contain antiseptic properties that are effective for both internal and external cleansing, and are beneficial for improving asthma, bronchitis, cholera and ear infections. They are also effective for cleaning toxins from the body and eliminating intestinal parasites. Even though lemons and limes are highly acidic upon consumption, they have an alkaline food ash after digestion and are extremely healthful. *Due to their initial acidic properties, citrus fruits should be avoided by those who suffer from arthritis, inflammation, gout or esophageal cancer.*

Mangoes – (vitamins A, B1, B2, B3, B5 & C, calcium, iron, magnesium, potassium, zinc)
Native to Southeast Asia and India, mangoes are considered to be the most widely consumed fresh fruit worldwide, and are loaded with potent antioxidants that assist a long list of health disorders. This sweet tasting fruit contains stomach-soothing digestive enzymes that help alleviate indigestion, irritable bowel syndrome, gallbladder disorders and peptic ulcers. Mangoes contain dietary fiber, are low in calories, and are an excellent food to replenish energy and body salts lost after exercise. They contain powerful antibacterial and antiviral properties that help protect against infections, inhibit the growth of tumors and reduce the risk of many forms of cancer. Mangoes also help to lower blood pressure and cholesterol levels, promote cardiovascular health, regulate blood sugar for diabetics and possess anti-inflammatory properties that help alleviate arthritis and gout. Because they are rich in iron, mangoes are beneficial for anemia and for women during pregnancy and menstruation. Additional benefits of this mouth-watering fruit include slowing premature aging, promoting healthy skin and relieving muscle cramps.

Mangosteen – (vitamins A, B1, B2, B3, C, D & E, calcium, folate, manganese, potassium, selenium)
Popular in Southeastern Asia for thousands of years, mangosteen is a tropical evergreen tree that yields a nutritious fruit containing *xanthones,* organic compounds that possess antibacterial, antifungal, antiviral and antiparasitic properties. Despite the similar name, this healthful fruit is not related to the mango, but has many similar health benefits. Mangosteen is an excellent source of antioxidants that help alleviate allergies, arthritis and inflammation, inhibit the growth of tumors which lowers the risk of cancer, and help slow down the aging process. It protects against obesity and fatigue by stimulating weight loss and providing a natural energy boost. Mangosteen has also been beneficial for easing anxiety and depression, reducing stomach ulcers, protecting against osteoporosis, and may even lower the risk of Alzheimer's and Parkinson's disease.

Mushrooms (*maitake, reishi, shiitake*) – (vitamins B1, B2, B3, B5 & C, copper, iron, protein)
Including shiitake, maitake and reishi, mushrooms have been used for years for their ability to stimulate and strengthen the immune system and ward off infectious diseases. They contain powerful antioxidants that have shown promise in reducing the risk of cancer, inhibiting tumor growth, lowering blood pressure and cholesterol levels and slowing the rate of cognitive decline. Considered a "Food of the Gods" by the ancient Romans, mushrooms contain antibacterial and antiviral properties that are effective against influenza. They also contain anti-inflammatory properties that have been effective for easing arthritis pain and alleviating asthma. Shiitake mushrooms contain a polysaccharide called *lentinan* that may help improve the immune system of people infected with HIV and AIDS. Mushrooms are excellent baked, braised, lightly grilled, roasted, steamed or lightly sautéed in olive oil and can be used in soups, salads, tonics, teas, herbal formulas and prepared foods.

Oats (*raw*) – (vitamin B1, manganese, phosphorous, selenium, protein)
Cultivated in Asia, Europe, Canada and North America, raw oats are a delicious, nutritious breakfast food that help improve cardiovascular health and are a great way to start your day! They are an excellent source of complex carbohydrates that are effective for stimulating metabolism, increasing energy, reducing obesity, and are rich in life-extending antioxidants. Oats are beneficial for lowering blood pressure and cholesterol levels, and improving digestive disorders such as constipation and irritable bowel syndrome. This amazing super food also protects against asthma, atherosclerosis, and may lower the risk of breast and colon cancer. Whole grains are rich in fiber and magnesium which are known to help lower the risk of Type 2 diabetes, and oats contain a specific type of soluble fiber called *beta-glucan* that has shown to stabilize blood sugar levels.

Olive Oil – (vitamin E, omega 9 fatty acid)
Dating as far back as 5000 B.C., this Mediterranean miracle known as extra virgin olive oil is a heart-smart, culinary oil rich in monounsaturated fats that provide powerful antioxidant benefits from vitamin E and various phytonutrients. Made from pressed olives, olive oil is a rich source of omega 9 fatty acids that promote cardiovascular health, protect against atherosclerosis and lower the risk of heart attack and stroke. Olive oil is known for protecting against many forms of cancer such as breast, colon, ovarian, pancreatic and prostate. It is also effective for restoring enzymes that neutralize toxins, controlling blood sugar, and lowering blood pressure and cholesterol levels. Additionally, olive oil promotes gastrointestinal health, protects against osteoporosis by preventing bone loss, and contains powerful anti-inflammatory properties that help alleviate asthma, bronchitis, arthritis and gout.

Onions – (vitamins B6 & C, dietary fiber, chromium, copper, folate, manganese, potassium)
Originally cultivated in Central Asia, the Middle East and parts of Russia, and enjoyed by the ancient Greeks and Romans, onions are one of the most popular and widely consumed foods in the world. This nutritious and flavorful vegetable contains powerful sulfur compounds that help protect against most forms of cancer. Related to scallions, shallots and leeks, onions contain antibacterial properties and a flavonoid called *quercitin* that is known to inhibit the growth of tumors. They are also beneficial for lowering blood pressure and cholesterol levels, preventing blood clot formation, protecting against atherosclerosis and reducing the risk of cardiovascular disease. Onions also contain anti-inflammatory compounds that help alleviate asthma, bronchitis, arthritis and gout, lower blood sugar and triglyceride levels and improve glucose tolerance for diabetics.

Oranges – (vitamins A, B1 & C, fiber, potassium)
Originating in China and introduced to Florida by Spanish explorers in the 16th century, oranges are a sweet, summer fruit rich in pectin, vitamin C and other powerful antioxidants that promote heart health. They contain every type of cancer inhibitor (beta-carotene, flavonoids and terpenes) and are associated with stopping cancer cells before they start to multiply. The nutrients in oranges also protect against premature aging, improve cardiovascular function, lower blood pressure and cholesterol levels, and help promote respiratory health by easing asthma and bronchitis. Furthermore, oranges are known for reducing the risk of breast, lung, prostate and stomach cancer, eliminating kidney stones, combating viral infections and strengthening the immune system.

Papayas – (vitamins A, C, E & K)
Considered the "fruit of the angels" by Christopher Columbus, papayas are rich in vitamin C, carotenes and other antioxidants that protect against premature aging, and have shown to reduce the risk of cervical, colon, lung, prostate and stomach cancer. This tropical fruit contains dietary fiber and an enzyme called *papain* that helps alleviate digestive disorders such as indigestion, irritable bowel syndrome, constipation and diarrhea. Papayas are effective at improving cardiovascular health, lowering blood pressure and cholesterol levels and protecting against atherosclerosis. They contain anti-inflammatory properties that help alleviate arthritis, asthma and bronchitis. Papayas are also beneficial for alkalizing the body's pH level, as well as improving the quality of blood cells, increasing blood platelet count and protecting against anemia. Additionally, papayas are beneficial for stimulating the immune system and promoting good vision by reducing the risk of cataracts and macular degeneration.

Peaches – (vitamins A, B1, B2, B3 & C, calcium, iron, phosphorous, potassium)

Native to China and relative of the apricot, peaches are a sweet and nutritious fruit that contain potent antioxidants which inhibit tumor growth and help slow down the effects of aging. They are rich in vitamin A and potassium which are known for alleviating asthma, bronchitis, inflammation and gout, and protecting against many forms of cancer. Peaches are beneficial for improving digestive health, correcting constipation, combating obesity and are beneficial for eliminating bladder and kidney stones. They are also effective at lowering blood pressure and cholesterol, alkalizing the body's pH level, and protecting against anemia. Additional benefits include reducing the risk of cataracts and macular degeneration, promoting healthy skin by reducing wrinkles and helping to eliminate intestinal parasites.

Pineapples – (vitamins B1, B6 & C, dietary fiber)

Originally cultivated in South America and now grown domestically in the tropical climate of Hawaii, pineapples are a nutritious fruit rich in *bromelain,* a powerful digestive enzyme that alleviates a number of digestive disorders and helps eliminate intestinal parasites. Available year round, pineapples are effective for alleviating arthritis and inflammation, lowering the risk of heart attack and stroke by dissolving blood clots, and are a great source of manganese which is beneficial for preventing osteoporosis and bone fractures. They contain antibacterial, antiviral and antioxidant properties that inhibit tumor growth and reduce the risk of many forms of cancer. Known for their tangy sweetness, mouth-watering pineapples are also beneficial for increasing energy, protecting against cataracts and macular degeneration and easing symptoms of menopause.

Pomegranates – (vitamins A, B6, C & E, calcium, iron, magnesium, phosphorus, potassium, zinc)

Dating back to ancient Greek civilization, pomegranates have been a widely revered food and are well known for their life-extending health benefits. They are loaded with powerful antioxidants that protect against cardiovascular disease, and remove toxins from our cells which helps prevent premature aging and the wrinkling of our skin. The nutrients found in pomegranates are known for reducing the risk of breast, lung and prostate cancer, are effective against atherosclerosis, and may even help slow the accumulation of plaque in the brain associated with Alzheimer's disease. Additionally, they are beneficial for lowering cholesterol levels, strengthening the immune system, reducing the risk of impotence, and contain anti-inflammatory properties that help alleviate arthritis and gout. Today, pomegranate juice is available as a tasty, heart-healthy beverage and is among the new favorites in the health food industry.

Prunes – (vitamin A, copper, dietary fiber, iron, potassium)

Chewy, rich-tasting prunes are dried plums that contain numerous vitamins and minerals that provide many nutritional benefits. They are loaded with antioxidants and phytonutrients called *phenols* that help neutralize cancer-causing toxins in the body. Prunes are beneficial for those who have anemia because they are a rich source of iron and contain various nutrients that assist in iron absorption. They have also been beneficial for alleviating arthritis, asthma, bronchitis and inflammation, controlling blood sugar levels and protecting against post-menopausal breast cancer. Prunes are a great source of dietary fiber that helps lower the risk of cardiovascular disease, protects against obesity and is effective at relieving constipation. They are also rich in potassium which lowers blood pressure and cholesterol levels, protects against atherosclerosis and helps lower the risk of osteoporosis.

Pumpkin Seeds – (vitamins C, E & K, copper, iron, magnesium, manganese, phosphorus, zinc)

Treasured by the Native Americans as both a nutritious food and an effective medicine, naturally flavored pumpkin seeds are rich in dietary fiber and are a crucial part of a healthy diet. Also known as *pepitas*, these flavorful seeds are available all year round and contain a myriad of heath-promoting properties. Pumpkin seeds contain zinc, carotenoids and other phytonutrients that help slow the multiplication of prostate cells which reduces the risk of BPH and prostate cancer. They are also known for reducing the risk of bladder, breast, colon, lung and skin cancer, strengthening the immune system and stimulating the production of detoxifying enzymes. Pumpkin seeds contain anti-inflammatory properties and are beneficial for alleviating arthritis, lowering blood pressure and cholesterol, protecting against sun damage and reducing the risk of osteoporosis by helping to maintain bone density. They are also extremely powerful in the elimination of tape worms and other intestinal parasites.

Quinoa – (vitamins B & E, copper, iron, magnesium, manganese, phosphorus, tryptophan)

Native to South America, quinoa was a staple food of the Incas and Aztecs, and today provides one of the highest quality proteins compared to most other grains. Containing all nine essential amino acids, quinoa is beneficial for lowering blood pressure and cholesterol, improving cardiovascular health, and has a low glycemic index (GI) score. It is effective for increasing energy and stamina, easing migraine headaches, and providing powerful antioxidant protection against cancer. One of the main ingredients in tabouli, quinoa is a complete protein similar to eggs and is a great substitute for pasta. It is commonly used in soups, salads and breakfast porridge, and is a great food option for post-menopausal women. Quinoa is "gluten-free" and is safe to eat for those who have Celiac disease. Other "gluten-free" grains include amaranth, brown rice, corn flour, flaxseed, millet and soy flour.

Raisins – (vitamin C, boron, calcium, iron, potassium)

Cultivated in Persia and Egypt around 2000 B.C., raisins are simply dehydrated grapes that contain powerful antioxidants and many health-promoting nutrients. Often referred to as "nature's candy," these high-energy, low-fat snacks are one of the richest food sources of *boron* that help lower the risk of osteoporosis, and are known to mimic the positive effects of estrogen therapy which may be beneficial for postmenopausal women. Raisins contain iron that assists in the formation of red blood cells, which is especially beneficial for pregnant women and those who suffer from anemia. They are also rich in dietary fiber which helps alleviate constipation, inhibits the growth of tumors and is powerful at protecting against colon and prostate cancer. Additionally, raisins are beneficial for reducing the risk of cataracts and macular degeneration, preventing gingivitis and tooth decay, increasing energy and are believed to stimulate the libido.

Salmon – (vitamins B3, B6, B12, D, tryptophan, protein)

Wild-caught salmon is one of the best sources of protein that nature provides, is low in calories and saturated fat, and is beneficial for heart health and proper brain function. It is rich in the omega-3 fatty acids *docosahexaenoic acid* (DHA) and *eicosapentaenoic acid* (EPA) which cannot be produced by the body, so it is necessary to get them from a food source. Regular consumption of salmon protects against cardiovascular disease, lung disease, osteoporosis and lupus and has even shown to improve conditions of depression. Additional benefits include alleviating arthritis, inflammation and gout, lowering blood pressure and cholesterol levels, promoting proper heart muscle function and preventing blood clots. Wild-caught salmon has minimal, if any, mercury content, and is believed to be a much healthier alternative over farmed salmon which often contains much higher levels of mercury. Shellfish are also abundant sources of protein and minerals, however because they are bottom feeders they may contain significant levels of mercury as well. **Pregnant women should avoid and/or use extreme caution when consuming any fish or fish oil supplements due to possible mercury content.*

Soy Foods – (vitamins A, B6, B12, C & D, calcium, protein)

The natural protein content in soy foods – including soybeans, soy milk, soy nuts, miso, tofu and tempeh – is equal to the protein quality of animal foods, which makes soy a nutritious meat substitute. They contain antioxidants, omega 3 & 6 fatty acids and have shown their ability for reducing tumor growth as well as lowering the risk of colon, lung, prostate, skin, stomach and testicular cancer. Soy foods are also known for protecting against kidney disorders and obesity as well as lowering blood pressure and cholesterol levels, improving cardiovascular health and strengthening the immune system. They are rich in phytoestrogens that mimic female hormones and have been linked to alleviating menopausal discomforts as well as reducing mood swings associated with PMS. The other side of soy is that soy foods may be hard to digest for some people, and may contain high levels of aluminum either absorbed from the soil or acquired from being processed on aluminum machinery. Not only does aluminum inhibit the absorption of zinc and other important minerals, it is thought to be the leading cause of Alzheimer's disease, senility and other various forms of dementia. To find aluminum-free soy products, *always* choose organic, read labels and research companies that do not use alkaline soaking solutions or aluminum equipment to produce their products.

Spinach – (vitamins A, B1, B2, B3, C, E & K, calcium, iron, magnesium, phosphorus, potassium)
Originally cultivated in Persia and utilized as a medicinal plant, spinach is a highly nutritious food rich in protein, antioxidants and fiber and is the most common food consumed by those who do not get cancer. This leafy green veggie contains over 12 different *flavonoid* compounds that inhibit tumor growth and help lower the risk of breast, colon, lung, ovarian, prostate, skin and stomach cancer. Loaded with vitamin K, folate and iron, spinach contains more nutrients than most other foods and is known for reducing the risk of cardiovascular disease, lowering blood pressure and cholesterol, protecting against osteoporosis and promoting proper brain function. It is beneficial for improving blood quality, increasing energy and vitality, and is a rich source of lutein which helps protect against cataracts and macular degeneration. Spinach contains anti-inflammatory properties that help alleviate asthma, bronchitis and migraine headaches; however, due to its high oxalic acid content, those who have arthritis and gout should consume spinach in moderation only.

Sweet Potatoes – (vitamins A, B6 & C, copper, dietary fiber, iron, manganese, potassium)
Native to Central America and consumed since the prehistoric ages, sweet potatoes are a tasty root vegetable that contains dietary fiber and powerful antioxidants that improve cardiovascular health and slow the effects of aging. Not to be confused with yams which are much lower in beta carotene, not as sweet-tasting and are mainly imported from the Caribbean, sweet potatoes are grown domestically, are an excellent source of beta carotene and come in a variety of colors such as orange, red, purple, white and yellow. Nutritionally superior to most other foods, sweet potatoes are associated with reducing the risk of colon, lung, prostate, skin and stomach cancer. They help protect against arthritis, inflammation, lower the risk of atherosclerosis, and are effective at alleviating constipation. Sweet potatoes are also beneficial for diabetics because they help stabilize blood sugar levels and improve insulin response.

Tomatoes – (vitamins A, B1, B3, B5, C, E & K, copper, iron, magnesium, phosphorous, potassium)
Native to Central and South America, tomatoes are a heart-healthy food rich in vitamin C and other powerful antioxidants that are effective at inhibiting tumor growth. These vine-ripened salad toppers are important for reducing the risk of most forms of cancer including bladder, breast, cervical, colon, lung, ovarian, pancreatic, prostate, skin, stomach and testicular. Tomatoes are a rich source of *lycopene,* a phytonutrient that not only reduces cell damage and helps protect our skin from the sun, but protects against cardiovascular disease and promotes healthy vision by lowering the risk of cataracts and macular degeneration. Available year round, they have also been effective for easing migraine headaches, promoting proper digestion, lowering blood pressure and cholesterol and protecting against diabetes by stabilizing blood sugar levels. Consuming tomatoes with olive oil helps increase the absorption of lycopene, and is believed to be one of the contributing factors of longevity associated with the Mediterranean diet.

Turkey – (vitamins B3 & B6, iron, protein, selenium, tryptophan, zinc)
A native dish of the United States and Mexico and synonymous with the Thanksgiving holiday, turkey is an excellent source of nutritious, low-fat protein that promotes cardiovascular health and strengthens the immune system. This highly palatable poultry is rich in amino acids and selenium that assist wound healing, support healthy thyroid function and help inhibit the growth of cancer cells. Turkey also contains vitamins B3 (niacin) & B6 (pyridoxine) that not only help the body covert protein into energy, but also help alleviate arthritis and inflammation, protect against senility and have shown promise in easing the symptoms of PMS. Tryptophan is an amino acid that is known for its sleep-inducing effects; however the myth with eating turkey and becoming sleepy is associated more with over-eating than its tryptophan content.

Watermelon – (vitamins A, B1, B6 & C, magnesium, potassium)
Enjoyed by ancient Egyptians as far back as 3000 B.C., watermelons are native to the Kalahari Desert of southern Africa and are loaded with dietary fiber, powerful antioxidants and other healthful nutrients that help lower blood pressure and cholesterol levels and neutralize harmful toxins. Like tomatoes, this sweet summer treat contains the phytonutrient *lycopene* that promotes cardiovascular health, strengthens the immune system, and reduces the risk of breast, cervical, colon, lung, ovarian, prostate, stomach and testicular cancer. Watermelon is a natural energy source rich in beta carotene that protects against cataracts and macular degeneration, reduces the risk of atherosclerosis, protects against erectile

dysfunction and helps improve skin disorders like eczema and psoriasis. This low-calorie, mouth-watering fruit not only quenches thirst, but also contains anti-inflammatory properties that help alleviate arthritis, asthma and bronchitis. Watermelons have a high glycemic Index (GI) score but are low in carbohydrates, so they have a lower glycemic load and do not spike blood sugar as much as similar high GI foods. Combining watermelon with protein and a healthy fat may help slow the absorption of sugar, however diabetics should only consume watermelon in moderation.

Yogurt – (vitamins B2, B5 & B12, calcium, iodine, potassium, zinc)
Consumed throughout the Middle East since the 13th century, yogurt is a high-quality complete protein that contains acidophilus, or 'friendly' bacteria cultures which strengthens the immune system, promotes gastrointestinal health, improves liver function and alleviates the effects of allergies. These active cultures in yogurt help improve digestive disorders such as colitis, flatulence and ulcers, protect against urinary tract and yeast infections, and may reduce the risk of colon cancer. Loaded with vitamins and minerals, this beneficial breakfast food has been effective for lowering blood pressure and LDL (bad) cholesterol levels while increasing HDL (good) cholesterol. Due to its high-calcium content, yogurt also promotes weight loss by burning belly fat, improves the body's recovery after a workout and greatly reduces the risk of osteoporosis. Organic low-fat or non-fat yogurt is a smart health option, and a nutritious dessert substitute for ice cream.

Zucchini – (vitamins A, B1, B2, B3, C & K, calcium, folate, magnesium, potassium, zinc)
Originally cultivated in southern Mexico and Central America, zucchini is a nutritious, cucumber-shaped vegetable that has been utilized for over 10,000 years for its nutritional benefits. Otherwise known as "summer squash," it comes in a variety of shapes, sizes, varieties and colors and is known to help protect against cardiovascular disease. Zucchini is loaded with antioxidants, omega 3's and powerful phytonutrients that help prevent the mutation of cancer cells. It has been effective for alleviating arthritis and asthma, lowering blood pressure and cholesterol levels, helping to reduce the risk of an enlarged prostate (Benign Prostatic Hypertrophy - BPH), and protecting against multiple sclerosis (MS). Zucchini is also rich in vitamin C which helps reduce bruising, and contains *lutein* which is necessary for proper vision and maintaining eye health.

Foods	Health Benefits			
Almonds	cardiovascular health	anti-aging properties	lowers cholesterol & blood pressure	beneficial for diabetes
Apples	improves lung function	stimulates weight loss	improves digestive disorders	cardiovascular health
Apricots	lowers cholesterol & blood pressure	reduces risk of anemia	promotes good vision	improves digestive disorders
Artichokes	improves liver function	stabilizes blood sugar	improves digestive disorders	lowers cholesterol & blood pressure
Avocados	lowers cholesterol & blood pressure	alleviates arthritis	cardiovascular health	promotes eye health
Bananas	protects against osteoporosis	normalizes blood pressure	eases arthritis & carpal tunnel	reduces risk of kidney cancer
Barley	lowers cholesterol & blood pressure	improves liver function	beneficial for diabetes	lowers risk of gallstones
Beans	stabilizes blood sugar	lowers cholesterol & blood pressure	anti-aging properties	helps prevent constipation
Beets	anti-cancer	reduces risk of neural tube defects	stabilizes blood sugar	protects against osteoporosis
Bell Peppers	respiratory health	lowers cholesterol & blood pressure	cardiovascular health	eases symptoms of menopause
Berries	anti-aging, anti-cancer	cardiovascular health	supports memory & good vision	beneficial for diabetes
Broccoli	anti-aging, anti-cancer	helps macular degeneration	lowers cholesterol & blood pressure	reduces risk of birth defects
Brown Rice	lowers cholesterol & blood pressure	supports healthy nervous system	improves digestive disorders	stimulates weight loss
Buckwheat	cardiovascular health	reduces risk of diabetes	helps eliminate gallstones	lowers cholesterol & blood pressure

Foods	Health Benefits			
Cabbage	anti-aging, anti-cancer	cardiovascular health	alleviates constipation	reduces risk of diabetes
Cantaloupe	lowers cholesterol & blood pressure	protects against kidney stones	promotes good vision	beneficial for obesity
Carrots	promotes good vision	anti-aging, anti-cancer	colitis & Crohn's disease	cardiovascular health
Cauliflower	detoxifies the body	cardiovascular health	improves liver function	reduces arthritis & inflammation
Celery	lowers cholesterol & blood pressure	reduces arthritis & inflammation	protects against osteoporosis	promotes blood clotting
Figs	protects against osteoporosis	normalizes metabolism	lowers cholesterol & blood pressure	cardiovascular health
Grapefruit	anti-cancer	strengthens the immune system	protects against kidney stones	lowers cholesterol & blood pressure
Grapes (red)	cardiovascular health	Alzheimer's disease	lowers cholesterol & blood pressure	reduces blood clots
Green Tea	anti-aging, anti-cancer	reduces risk of prostate cancer	stabilizes blood sugar	lowers cholesterol & blood pressure
Honey (raw)	antibacterial, antiviral	lowers cholesterol & blood pressure	helps muscles recuperate	stabilizes blood sugar
Kale	anti-cancer	slows mental decline	reduces arthritis & inflammation	macular degeneration
Kelp	anti-cancer	stimulates thyroid function	protects against radiation	beneficial for spinal cord
Lemons/Limes	strengthens the immune system	cardiovascular health	helps eliminate intestinal parasites	alleviates asthma & bronchitis
Mangoes	lowers cholesterol & blood pressure	promotes good vision	antibacterial, antiviral	healthy skin & teeth

Foods	Health Benefits			
Mangosteen	reduces arthritis & inflammation	anti-aging, anti-cancer	beneficial for obesity	lowers cholesterol & blood pressure
Mushrooms	strengthens the immune system	lowers cholesterol & blood pressure	supports kidney & liver health	reduces arthritis & inflammation
Oats (raw)	reduces risk of atherosclerosis	eases fatigue & depression	lowers cholesterol & blood pressure	normalizes metabolism
Olive Oil	gallbladder, liver & kidney health	improves digestive disorders	stabilizes blood sugar	lowers cholesterol & blood pressure
Onions	anti-cancer & anti-tumor	stabilizes blood sugar	lowers cholesterol & blood pressure	cardiovascular health
Oranges	cardiovascular health	strengthens the immune system	protects against kidney stones	alleviates asthma & bronchitis
Papayas	promotes good vision	reduces arthritis & inflammation	improves digestive disorders	strengthens the immune system
Peaches	lowers cholesterol & blood pressure	promotes good vision	improves lung function	improves digestive disorders
Pineapples	reduces arthritis & inflammation	improves digestive disorders	protects against osteoporosis	anti-parasitic
Pomegranates	anti-aging, anti-cancer	Alzheimer's disease	reduces arthritis & inflammation	strengthens the immune system
Prunes	improves digestive disorders	stimulates energy & weight loss	good for PMS & breast cancer	lowers cholesterol & blood pressure
Pumpkin Seeds	lower risk of prostate cancer	lowers cholesterol & blood pressure	anti-parasitic	reduces arthritis & inflammation
Quinoa	lowers cholesterol & blood pressure	beneficial for diabetes	cardiovascular health	eases migraines
Raisins	lower risk of prostate cancer	healthy teeth & gums	protects against osteoporosis	promotes good vision

Foods	Health Benefits			
Salmon	cardiovascular health	lowers cholesterol & blood pressure	reduces blood clots	improves lung function
Soy Foods	anti-aging, anti-cancer	cardiovascular health	lowers cholesterol & blood pressure	strengthens the immune system
Spinach	supports brain function	anti-aging, anti-cancer	protects against osteoporosis	lowers cholesterol & blood pressure
Sweet Potatoes	protects against colon cancer	reduces arthritis & inflammation	improves lung function	improves digestive disorders
Tomatoes	lower risk of prostate cancer	promotes good vision	lowers cholesterol & blood pressure	stabilizes blood sugar
Turkey	cardiovascular health	eases symptoms of PMS	strengthens the immune system	reduces arthritis & inflammation
Watermelon	colon & prostate health	reduces arthritis & inflammation	promotes good vision	lowers cholesterol & blood pressure
Yogurt	protects against osteoporosis	lowers cholesterol & blood pressure	reduces yeast infections	strengthens the immune system
Zucchini	reduces risk of prostate cancer	combats (MS) multiple sclerosis	alleviates arthritis & asthma	lowers cholesterol & blood pressure

~ Natural Supplements ~

Aloe Vera Juice – (vitamins A, B1, B2, B6, B12, C & E, calcium, magnesium, sodium, zinc)
For thousands of years, the aloe vera plant has been used to improve skin conditions, as a remedy for sunburns and as a natural moisturizer. It has also been used to alleviate acne, blemishes, burns, cuts, insect stings, infections, skin cancer and other dermatologic disorders. Unknown to many people, pure aloe vera juice is a remarkable, natural health supplement with countless health benefits when taken internally. It is sugar free and contains various vitamins, minerals phytonutrients and amino acids necessary for optimal health. Aloe vera juice has been used for lowering cholesterol levels, alleviating arthritis and inflammation, controlling blood sugar and increasing energy. It is effective for improving lung function, and has shown promise in protecting against lung cancer. This natural remedy contains antibacterial, antifungal and antiviral properties, increases white blood cell count, strengthens the immune system, and may be beneficial for those who have HIV. Aloe vera juice helps improve digestive disorders such as colitis, heartburn, irritable bowel syndrome, indigestion, hemorrhoids and ulcers. Aging increases the acidity of our bodies, and most of the common ailments we suffer from can only thrive in an acidic body state. Since aloe vera juice is alkaline, it helps restore the body back to its proper pH level, is extremely effective against acidosis and premature aging, and protects against many forms of cancer. Additional benefits include stimulating cell regeneration, detoxifying the organs and bloodstream, and increasing circulation in the extremities. This is one powerful weapon in the arsenal of natural health!

Apple Cider Vinegar – (vitamins A, B1, B2, C & E, calcium, magnesium, potassium, sulfur, zinc)
Utilized by the ancient Egyptians around 3000 BC, apple cider vinegar is a powerful detoxifying supplement that has been beneficial for improving a long list of health disorders. High-quality vinegar will be organic, unfiltered with a brownish hue and contain many beneficial nutrients. Apple cider vinegar is one of the richest sources of amino acids known, and helpful for alleviating allergies, improving memory and protecting the mind from various forms of dementia such as senility and Alzheimer's disease. During the U.S. Civil War and World War I, apple cider vinegar was used to clean the wounds of injured soldiers. It is also beneficial for normalizing digestive disorders like constipation and irritable bowel syndrome, improving various skin disorders such as eczema and psoriasis, and alleviating migraine headaches. Apple cider vinegar helps reduce the effects of food poisoning,

improves bacterial, fungal, viral and yeast infections, and is powerful against pneumonia. It has also been effective for alleviating arthritis and inflammation, lowering blood pressure and cholesterol, and stimulating weight loss by breaking down fats. Even though apple cider vinegar is acidic before ingested, it has an alkaline food ash after digestion which helps reduce acidity in the body.

Bentonite – (calcite, feldspar, gypsum, magnesium, quartz)

Bentonite (*montmorillonite*) is a natural clay mineral created from the residue of weathered volcanic ash, and contains over 70 trace minerals, and is beneficial for detoxifying the body and increasing the absorption of nutrients. Ancient civilizations like the Indians of the high Andes, the aborigines of Australia and various tribes in Africa have used bentonite clay to improve intestinal disorders and detoxify the body. It is able to absorb free radicals like a sponge which makes it one of the most effective, naturally detoxifying substances available. Bentonite's ability to bind and neutralize toxins has an electrical aspect to it; minerals are negatively charged while toxins are positively charged so the clay's attraction is magnetic and draws toxins to it. The clay contains fine molecules that have a greater surface area which gives it stronger absorbing or pulling power. Bentonite is also an effective colon and liver cleanser, protects against cirrhosis and hepatitis, and improves various digestive disorders such as constipation, diarrhea and irritable bowel syndrome. This volcanic detoxifier helps the body recover from radiation therapy, is excellent for eliminating intestinal parasites, and will actually pass through the body undigested. Bentonite is most effective taken on an empty stomach or a couple hours after meals.

Brewer's Yeast – (vitamins B1, B2, B3, B6, B9, B12, chromium, copper, selenium, zinc)

Brewer's yeast is collected as a by-product of the beer brewing process, yet is well known to have a wide range of health benefits. It is loaded with 16 amino acids, B vitamins, minerals, protein and is low in calories, carbohydrates, fat and sodium. Brewer's yeast has been known to help improve conditions such as anemia, eczema, anxiety and fatigue, as well as relieving constipation, lowering cholesterol and reducing stress. It is also a rich source of chromium; an essential trace mineral the body needs in order to regulate blood sugar levels. Brewer's yeast can be added to foods like pasta, stews, rice dishes, potatoes and meats, but should be added towards the end because the cooking process may destroy its nutritional content. **Due to possible allergic reactions, it is extremely important for diabetics to consult their doctor before consuming brewer's yeast.*

Calcium (*chelated*)

Calcium is the single most abundant and important mineral in the human body, but is the most difficult for the body to absorb. As we get older our bodies absorb less calcium when it is needed the most. When the body lacks calcium it is taken directly from the bones which may lead to osteoporosis and a number of other physiological disorders. Chelation is a process of binding molecules together to increase nutrient absorption, which is why *chelated* calcium is such an asset to preventative health. Obtaining calcium from food sources like broccoli, cheese, milk, spinach and yogurt is always ideal, but adding a high-quality calcium supplement to the diet can be a tremendous health advantage. Calcium is not only important for strong bones and healthy skin, but also for proper muscle growth, normalizing heart rhythm, for the transmission of nerve impulses and many other important roles on the cellular level. It is also effective for alleviating arthritis, asthma, tendon and muscle pain, stimulating weight loss and promoting proper blood clotting. Two key factors to consider when buying calcium supplements are the type of calcium, and amount of elemental calcium they contain. Calcium citrate is a form of chelated calcium and is absorbed more quickly than calcium carbonate. However, calcium carbonate usually contains more elemental calcium than calcium citrate so it is important to read nutritional labels. The human body can absorb about 600 milligrams of elemental calcium at a time, so spreading out calcium intake helps increase absorption. Taking a calcium supplement before bed is ideal as this further increases assimilation and induces sleep. The nutrients that are needed for proper calcium absorption include essential fatty acids, vitamins A, C, D & E, boron, magnesium, manganese & phosphorus. **Iron supplements interfere with calcium absorption so it is best to take them separately. Whole grains contain a substance called phytic acid that binds to calcium and prevents its absorption, so they should be consumed at different times.*

Chia Seeds – (vitamins A, all B vitamins, C, D, E & K, boron, calcium, copper, iron, potassium, zinc)

As far back as 3000 BC, chia seeds were a staple food of the Mayans, Aztecs and Native American tribes, and were used for their amazing ability to increase energy and endurance. Known as the 'running food', they provide more nutrients for fewer calories than almost any other food and are gluten-free. Loaded with omega-3 fatty acids, chia seeds contain more protein than salmon and help to alleviate arthritis and inflammation, improve brain function and promote muscle growth. These tiny seeds are an excellent source of vitamins, minerals and phytonutrients, and are beneficial for cardiovascular, liver, breast and prostate health. Chia seeds provide soluble and insoluble fiber that improves digestive regularity, and lowers blood pressure and cholesterol levels. They also help control blood sugar levels by slowing down how fast our bodies convert carbohydrates into sugar, and are therefore beneficial for those who have Type 2 diabetes. Many use chia seeds for weight loss, as they seem to help reduce food cravings and create the feeling of being full. When mixed with water or ingested, they expand and form a bulky 'chia gel' around the outside of the seed, absorbing up to 10 times their weight in water. Chia seeds are especially popular with athletes because they keep them well hydrated, increase endurance and balance electrolytes. They have a nutty flavor and can be enjoyed with cereal, yogurt, on salads or baked in breads. Who knew the little seeds from the 70's chia pet toy we grew up with were such a revered, nutritional powerhouse? Ch-Ch-Ch-Chia!

Coconut Oil – (vitamins A, B2, B3, B6, B12, E & K, iron)

Native to the Caribbean, Hawaii, India, Malaysia, Polynesia, Asia, the South Pacific islands, South America and Florida, coconuts are packed full of life-extending nutrients. They were once so valuable to their cultivators that they were actually traded as currency in the 16th century. The fruit of the coconut is consumed as food, milk, oil, sugar and water, and has long been a nutritional staple of these tropical civilizations. Coconut oil is made up of 90% saturated fats, but they are medium chain triglycerides so they assimilate better. It contains fewer calories than other oils so it converts into energy easier and does not accumulate in the arteries. Many nutritional benefits have been linked to the antioxidants and *lauric acid* in virgin coconut oil such as helping to normalize blood pressure and cholesterol, reducing the risk of cancer, improving kidney disorders, preventing premature aging and increasing bone strength. The antibacterial, antifungal and antiviral properties of coconut oil also protect against herpes, influenza, strengthen the immune system, and may help reduce the viral susceptibility to HIV. Additional benefits include easing digestive disorders such as irritable bowel syndrome and indigestion, stimulating weight loss, increasing energy, reducing stress, and improving skin, hair and dental health. Mahalo!

CoQ10 – (coenzyme Q10)

CoQ10 is one of the most effective antioxidants that protects the heart, strengthens the immune system and reduces free radical damage to the cells. This life-extending nutrient, found in its greatest concentration in the heart, exists in high levels when we are born. The amount of CoQ10 in our bodies is at its peak when we are in our mid twenties and is what helps us look and stay young. However, these levels decline with age, so it's important to understand its significance as it is among the most powerful anti-aging supplements available. CoQ10 is one of the main nutrients our bodies need to produce physical energy, provides much needed energy for the heart to pump blood through the body, and helps strengthen the heart muscle. It improves cardiovascular health, protects against cancer, helps lower blood pressure and cholesterol levels, and is believed to reduce the risk of senility and Alzheimer's disease. CoQ10 has also been used for improving infertility, easing headaches, and is an excellent supplement for detoxifying the body on the cellular level.

Cordyceps – (adenosine, mannitol (cordycepic acid), polysaccharides)
Native to Nepal, Tibet and provinces of the Himalayas, Cordyceps are an extremely rare medicinal mushroom that has been used in Traditional Chinese Medicine for over 5,000 years. Also known as the "Chinese Mushroom," or "Caterpillar Mushroom" here in North America, this famous fungus was once only available to Chinese emperors and the very wealthy. Cordyceps are known for strengthening the immune system, improving adrenal function, lowering blood pressure and cholesterol, preventing kidney disease, and protecting against liver disorders such as hepatitis and cirrhosis. Containing powerful antioxidants, they are known for substantially reducing the risk of infections, tumors and certain forms of cancer including colon, lung and stomach. Cordyceps have been used by various athletes to increase blood flow and oxygen supplies to the body. It helps improve lung function, increases energy levels, enhances athletic performance and endurance, and promotes muscle growth. Cordyceps are also beneficial for improving glucose metabolism beneficial for diabetics, to improve impotence and infertility, and as a powerful aphrodisiac to enhance the libido. **Cordyceps should not be taken by those who have bladder, breast, ovarian or prostate cancer.*

Echinacea – (vitamins B1, B2, B3 & C, calcium, magnesium, phosphorus, potassium, selenium, zinc)
One of the most effective and respected herbal supplements today, echinacea has been used for hundreds of years to help alleviate coughing and sore throats, colds, fevers and the flu. Echinacea is most widely revered for its ability to stimulate the immune system by effectively strengthening white blood cells. It helps protect against disorders like meningitis, urinary tract and yeast infections, detoxifies both circulatory and respiratory systems, and contains powerful antioxidants that protect against premature aging. Echinacea also provides antibiotic benefits when applied topically, helps reduce infections and wounds, and improves skin disorders like acne, boils, eczema and psoriasis.

Fish Oil – (vitamin B6, copper, folate, magnesium, manganese, phosphorus)
Fish oil supplements contain both omega-3 essential fatty acids DHA and EPA which strengthens cardiovascular health, alleviates arthritis and inflammation and lowers blood pressure and cholesterol

levels. It contains powerful anti-aging properties that help increase longevity, improve skin disorders and promote eye health. Fish oil is a potent anti-cancer supplement that is beneficial for inhibiting the growth of tumors, as well as controlling blood sugar levels, reducing anxiety and depression, and protecting against senility and Alzheimer's disease. Similar to salmon, other quality food sources of omega 3 fish oil include albacore tuna, herring, mackerel, sardines, swordfish and trout. Due to its higher content of omega 3's, fish oil provides similar yet more compelling nutritional benefits than the alpha-linolenic acid (ALA) found in flaxseed oil. Cod liver oil contains omega-3 fatty acids as fish oil, plus significant levels of vitamins A and D which help protect against breast, colon and prostate cancer. However, exceeding the recommended daily allowance (RDA) of vitamin A may become harmful and has been associated with birth defects. Both fish and cold liver oils may contain toxins such as mercury and polychlorinated biphenyls (PCB's), so be diligent when adding this supplement to any diet. Many fish oil products are purified through a distillation process, so reading product labels to make sure you are getting a high-quality supplement is important.

Flaxseed Oil – (vitamin B6, copper, folate, magnesium, manganese, phosphorus, potassium, zinc)
Flaxseed oil is a natural substance derived from the flaxseed and is essential for a heart-healthy life. It is the richest plant source of omega-3's, and also contains omega-6 and omega-9 essential fatty acids (EFA's) which are necessary for improving memory, moods, concentration and for proper brain function. EFA's are the main components in flaxseeds that efficiently work throughout the body to protect cells from damaging substances while admitting healthy ones. Flaxseed oil is also the richest source of *lignans,* a fiber compound found in plants that lowers blood pressure, cholesterol and triglyceride levels, and helps clean the arteries of plaque which reduces the risk of atherosclerosis. It contains the omega 3 alpha-linolenic fatty acid (ALA) which improves cardiovascular health, stabilizes blood sugar levels, has antibacterial, antifungal and antiviral properties, and helps reduce the risk of colon cancer. It contains approximately 50% more omega 3's than fish oil, but does not contain any of the beneficial DHA or EPA fatty acids abundant in fish oil. Additionally, flaxseed oil helps alleviate pain and inflammation from arthritis, improves eyesight and the perception of colors, normalizes liver function and promotes strong bones, nails, skin and teeth. The proteins in flaxseed oil are easily digested, and contain important amino acids that the body requires for proper function. They protect against harmful toxin damage, reduce excess stomach acid and relieve symptoms of heartburn, indigestion and irritable bowel syndrome. For vegetarians, flaxseed oil is a great source of natural protein used as a nutritious substitute for fish oil.

Ginkgo Biloba – (vitamins A, B1, B2, B3 & C, calcium, magnesium, phosphorus, potassium, zinc)
Dating back to the Jurassic era and once thought to be extinct, ginkgo biloba is a rare type of tree native to China that for centuries has been utilized for its various health benefits. It is most widely known and revered for improving the effects of senility, increasing memory and promoting proper brain function. Ginkgo biloba helps reduce muscle cramps from clogged arteries, and protects against impotence by increasing circulation and tissue oxygenation. It contains powerful antioxidant properties that are beneficial for easing asthma and bronchitis, alleviating headaches and migraines, and may be effective in reducing the risk of senility and Alzheimer's disease. Ginkgo biloba is also known to protect against kidney disorders, improve conditions of eczema, increase energy and help ease depression. Other benefits include alleviating altitude sickness, reducing PMS discomforts and protecting organs against radiation damage. **Ginkgo biloba should not be used if there is a lack of blood clotting ability, before surgery or before any type of dental procedure.*

Ginseng – (vitamins B1, B2, B3, B9 & C, calcium, iron, magnesium, phosphorus, potassium, zinc)
Native to Asia and Siberia, ginseng has been revered for thousands of years in Traditional Chinese Medicine for its ability to promote proper adrenal function, alleviate symptoms of PMS as well as many other disorders. It is beneficial for relieving anxiety, depression, mood swings and stress, and increasing mental alertness. This nutritious spice is well known for increasing testosterone levels, sperm production and reducing the risk of erectile dysfunction. Ginseng has been effective for stimulating both the immune and nervous systems, inhibiting the growth of cancer cells, lowering blood pressure and cholesterol levels and relieving symptoms of the flu and common cold. It is rich in folate which increases the production of red blood cells, and improves digestive disorders such as diarrhea, indigestion and ulcers. Ginseng increases circulation and athletic endurance, reduces fatigue, and is beneficial for obesity because it is a natural appetite suppressant. It is also effective for lowering blood sugar levels for diabetics, and may help reduce the risk of Alzheimer's disease. Additional benefits include alleviating arthritis, inflammation, asthma and bronchitis. **Ginseng should not be used by those who have high blood pressure or insomnia.*

Grape Seed Extract – (vitamin E, flavonoids, linoleic acid, resveratrol)
Grape seed extract is a liquid derivative of the grape seed and is one of the most powerful antioxidants nature provides. Belonging to a class of phytonutrients called *bioflavonoids,* it has been effective for lowering blood pressure and cholesterol levels, improving cardiovascular health and protecting against

premature aging. Grape seed extract is especially beneficial for athletes because it binds to collagen fibers increasing muscle flexibility and strengthening the elasticity of ligaments and tendons. This nutrient-dense supplement protect cells from toxins caused by pollution, smoking, stress and other environmental factors. Grape seed extract increases circulation, helps reduce the formation of plaque in the arteries, and is beneficial for those who suffer from dementia because it increases mental alertness. It is also effective for alleviating arthritis and inflammation, reducing the risk of most forms of cancer (except bladder), and may help protect against Parkinson's disease. Furthermore, grape seed extract supports liver and kidney health, improves digestive function, promotes eye health and helps eliminate bacterial and viral infections.

Graviola – (vitamins B1, B2 & C)

Graviola is a small evergreen tree that is native to South America and the Amazon jungle, as well as tropical areas of Central America and throughout the Caribbean. In the Amazon rainforest, every part of the Graviola tree, including the bark, fruits, leaves, roots and seeds is utilized. Graviola has been used to improve a variety of health disorders including arthritis, asthma, bronchitis, inflammation, liver disorders and for lowering blood pressure and cholesterol levels. It has been effective for strengthening the immune system, protecting against bacterial and viral infections, reducing colds, fever and the flu and improving insomnia. Graviola contains a powerful phytonutrient called *annonaceous acetogenins* that is known to inhibit the growth of tumors, and reduce the risk of many forms of cancer including breast, colon, lung, pancreatic and prostate. It has also been known for effectively eliminating intestinal parasites, head lice, skin aliments, and for improving conditions of colitis and diarrhea. Additionally, graviola improves digestion, relieves nausea, and helps increase blood flow by dilating blood vessels. **Graviola contains alkaloids and should be avoided by those who have Parkinson's disease.*

Lecithin – (vitamins B1, B2 & C)

A brow-yellowish fatty substance naturally occurring in animal and plant tissues, egg yolks and soy beans, lecithin plays an important role in optimizing health. It stimulates weight loss by breaking down fats in the body, and helps prevent fat accumulation in the liver which protects against cirrhosis and hepatitis. Lecithin is extremely important for managing the flow of nutrients and waste materials in and out of cells. It is beneficial for lowering blood pressure and cholesterol levels, improving cardiovascular health, and reducing the risk of atherosclerosis by protecting against plaque build up in the arteries. Along with its main component choline, lecithin is known for improving women's reproductive health, supporting a healthy pregnancy, promoting proper infant growth, sustaining healthy breast cells and easing the discomforts of menopause. Lecithin is also beneficial for men's reproductive health because it is a major component of sperm, and soy lecithin supplements have been found to increase the volume of prostate secretions. Furthermore, it is beneficial for fibromyalgia and multiple sclerosis (MS), protects against gallstones and pancreatitis, helps alleviate narcolepsy and improves psoriasis. Last but not least, lecithin is effective for improving brain function and may help reduce the risk of dementia.

Milk Thistle – (calcium, iron, magnesium, manganese, phosphorus, potassium, selenium, zinc)
Milk thistle has been used for thousands of years to improve a variety of disorders, but is especially known for its positive effects on the liver. It contains powerful antioxidants that help normalize enzyme levels, and protects the liver and kidneys from damage caused by alcohol, environmental toxins, viruses and over-the-counter pain relievers such as acetaminophen and ibuprofen. The liver is the 2nd largest organ and acts as a filter for cleaning toxins out of our bodies. Milk thistle contains *silymarin*, a natural substance known to help regenerate damaged liver cells and tissues, and is especially important for those with cirrhosis or hepatitis. It is beneficial for strengthening the immune system, reducing the risk of atherosclerosis, and protecting against bladder, breast, colon, lung and prostate cancer. Milk thistle is also effective for normalizing metabolism, improving adrenal, digestive and gallbladder function, increasing the absorption of nutrients and maintaining healthy blood quality. Additionally, it enables the liver to process estrogen more effectively which helps women who suffer from infertility. Many athletes and bodybuilders who use performance-enhancing supplements like anabolic steroids, prohormones, and thermogenics also use milk thistle to reduce stress on the liver.

Psyllium – (calcium, dietary fiber, potassium)
Psyllium is a natural grain extracted from the husks of the psyllium seed that provides extensive cardiovascular benefits. It is most commonly used for its dietary fiber content and strong laxative effects, and is the active ingredient in Metamucil. Psyllium is a water-soluble fiber that reduces the risk of colon cancer. It cleans the entire digestive system by eliminating toxins, heavy metals and excess waste from the body. Psyllium is effective for lowering blood pressure and cholesterol levels, and reducing the risk of heart attack and stroke. It is also beneficial for relieving constipation, increasing energy, and stimulates a sluggish metabolism caused by poor nutrition, lack of exercise and excessive stress from fast-paced lifestyles. Containing no sugar, salt or preservatives, psyllium is very easy on the digestive system, and helps control blood sugar levels which is especially important for those with diabetes. Psyllium expands quickly when mixed with water and should be consumed immediately!

Royal Jelly – (vitamins B5, B6 & C, collagen, zinc)

Royal jelly is a milky substance secreted from young worker bees between their 6th and 12th days of life. When these special nurse bees combine honey and pollen, they naturally create royal jelly. Rich in DNA, RNA, enzymes, hormones, protein, vitamins and minerals, royal jelly acts as a catalyst for cell regeneration, contains powerful anti-aging and anti-tumor properties and helps strengthen the immune system. It is a rich source of collagen and zinc which protects against osteoporosis by enhancing the formation of bone tissue, and contains the compound (10H2DA) that has shown to inhibit joint destruction beneficial for those who suffer from arthritis, inflammation and gout. Royal jelly increases red blood cell count, improves blood quality beneficial for those who are anemic, and protects against atherosclerosis by helping to prevent the narrowing of the arteries. It is beneficial for lowering cholesterol, and is a great source of glucose and fructose which helps stabilize blood-sugar levels. Loaded with amino acids and various phytonutrients, royal jelly helps protect against autoimmune disorders such as lupus, fibromyalgia, multiple sclerosis (MS) and Parkinson's disease. It provides protection against liver disorders like cirrhosis and hepatitis, enhances sexual vitality, increases energy, and is one of the most effective carbohydrates to take before exercise. Royal jelly is a great source of cancer-fighting antioxidants, and is beneficial for alleviating anxiety, depression, migraine headaches, as well as protecting against various forms of dementia. Possessing antibacterial, antifungal and antiviral properties, royal jelly also protects against various skin disorders like acne, eczema, canker sores and mouth ulcers.

Saw Palmetto – (beta carotene, fatty acids, tannins)

Saw palmetto is a small palm-type shrub native to the Atlantic and Gulf coastal plains, and is also grown in southern Europe and Africa as well. The dark purple-colored fruit from this tree was used by Native Americans to improve a variety of digestive and genital disorders. Increasingly popular in Europe, this herbal extract is used as an antiseptic, diuretic, expectorant, sedative, for easing menstrual discomforts and as a tonic for soothing the digestive tract. Saw Palmetto is known to lower the risk of prostate cancer by its ability to shrink the prostate gland and inhibit cancerous cell growth within the inner lining of the prostate. It helps suppress the production of *dihydrotestosterone* (DHT), a form of testosterone the body produces that causes enlargement of the prostate gland. Saw palmetto contains fatty acids that help alleviate symptoms of testicular and urinary inflammation, support healthy hormone levels, protect against impotence and infertility, increase sexual stamina and may be beneficial for improving male pattern baldness. **Saw Palmetto contains a substance similar to cholesterol called beta-sitosterol and should be avoided by those who have high cholesterol or poor cardiovascular health.*

Spirulina – (vitamins B1, B2, B3, C & E, calcium, chromium, magnesium, potassium, selenium, zinc) Thriving in hot climates around the world, spirulina is a microalgae consisting of vegetable proteins, chlorophyll, dietary fiber and many other healthful nutrients. It contains more beta carotene than carrots, a higher concentration of protein than soybeans, and contains a rare fatty acid called *gamma-linolenic acid* (GLA). This fatty acid is found in mother's milk and is essential for the proper development of healthy babies. Spirulina is rich in amino acids, B vitamins, various minerals and other essential nutrients that help reduce the risk of cancer, lower blood pressure and cholesterol, strengthen the immune system and help protect against anemia. An excellent source of natural energy, it promotes healthy nerves and tissues, increases nutrient absorption and helps detoxify the kidneys. Spirulina may also be beneficial for those who are diabetic or hypoglycemic, because it helps stabilize blood sugar levels when taken between meals.

St. John's Wort – (vitamin C, fatty acids, tannins)
Native to Asia, Europe and North America, St. John's wort was utilized for thousands of years for improving a variety of disorders like bruising, burns, dermatitis, diarrhea and jaundice. It is most commonly used as an anti-depressant and to reduce stress, but is also effective for relieving urinary tract infections, supporting the immune system and contains antiviral properties which may be beneficial for those with HIV & AIDS. Rich in phytonutrients, St. John's wort protects bone marrow from radiation damage, reduces swelling of the tendons and helps relieve pain associated with carpal tunnel syndrome (CTS). Excellent when seeped as a tea, St. John's wort is effective against tooth decay, and contains antibiotic properties that help alleviate bronchitis, congestion, phlegm, sinus infections and ulcers. **St. John's wort may produce side effects when combined with medications or asthma inhalers, and should be avoided by those who have dementia.*

Wheatgrass Juice – (vitamins A, C & E, calcium, iron, magnesium, phosphorus, potassium, protein)
Wheatgrass juice is considered the nectar of life, and is one of the most important nutritional supplements available. Green drinks are rich in vitamins, minerals, enzymes, antioxidants, provide phytonutrients to every cell in the body, protect our DNA and contain powerful anti-aging properties. Chlorophyll is the green pigment found in plants, the first product of light and contains more light energy than any other element. Wheatgrass juice is about 70% chlorophyll and is an excellent blood cleanser. The molecular structure of chlorophyll resembles that of the oxygen-carrying protein of red blood cells hemoglobin, and is considerably adaptable to our blood. The human body functions best

when it is highly oxygenated. Wheatgrass juice is rich in oxygen, and increases the amount of oxygen in the bloodstream which improves cardiovascular health. It is beneficial for anemia, helps control blood sugar levels and detoxifies the kidneys and liver. Wheatgrass juice is effective for lowering blood pressure and cholesterol, protecting against most forms of cancer (except pancreatic), and provides a natural energy boost. It helps restore vitality by removing heavy metals like lead, mercury and arsenic from the body, and is believed to help slow the process of graying hair. Additional benefits include alleviating arthritis and inflammation, reducing inner ear infections, cleaning the lymph system and protecting against tooth decay. Wheatgrass juice is also effective for improving infections, wounds, ulcers and tumors, as well as skin disorders such as acne, eczema and psoriasis.

Supplements	Health Benefits			
Aloe Vera Juice	eases digestive disorders	reduces arthritis & inflammation	beneficial for HIV & AIDS	protects against tumors & ulcers
Apple Cider Vinegar	lowers cholesterol & blood pressure	beneficial for eczema/psoriasis	reduces arthritis & inflammation	good for senility & Alzheimer's
Bentonite	eliminates toxins	beneficial for hepatitis	antiparasitic properties	digestive disorders
Brewer's Yeast	lowers cholesterol	stabilizes blood sugar	alleviates constipation	reduces fatigue
Calcium (chelated)	reduces risk of osteoporosis	supports nervous system health	eases tendon & muscle pain	promotes proper blood clotting
Chia Seeds	increases energy & endurance	lowers cholesterol	reduces arthritis & inflammation	stabilizes blood sugar
Coconut Oil	strengthens the immune system	anti-cancer	digestive disorders	beneficial for HIV & AIDS
CoQ10	anti-aging, anti-cancer	lowers cholesterol & blood pressure	increases energy	protects against Alzheimer's
Cordyceps	promotes liver & kidney health	increases energy	improves adrenal function	strengthens the immune system
Echinacea	strengthens the immune system	antibacterial, antiviral	detoxifies the body	beneficial for lymphatic system
Fish Oil	cardiovascular health	lowers cholesterol & blood pressure	reduces arthritis & inflammation	protects against diabetes
Flaxseed Oil	lowers cholesterol & blood pressure	improves liver function	cardiovascular health	reduces arthritis & inflammation

Supplements	Health Benefits			
Ginkgo Biloba	circulation & brain function	good for senility & Alzheimer's	eases migraine headaches	reduces risk of impotence
Ginseng	supports adrenal function	immune system, nervous system	helps reduce colds & the flu	eases PMS symptoms
Grape Seed Extract	good for senility & Alzheimer's	promotes liver & kidney health	reduces arthritis & inflammation	anti-aging properties
Graviola	antibacterial, antiviral	lowers cholesterol & blood pressure	intestinal parasites	reduces arthritis & inflammation
Lecithin	stimulates weight loss	cirrhosis & hepatitis	good for senility & Alzheimer's	reduces risk of gallstones
Milk Thistle	promotes liver & kidney health	strengthens the immune system	increases nutrient absorption	adrenal & gallbladder health
Pysllium	helps alleviate constipation	lowers cholesterol & blood pressure	reduces risk of colon cancer	detoxifies the body
Royal Jelly	increases red blood cells	reduces risk of atherosclerosis	cirrhosis & hepatitis	reduces risk of osteoporosis
Saw Palmetto	reduces risk of prostate cancer	alleviates urinary inflammation	eases symptoms of PMS	improves infertility & impotence
Spirulina	supports healthy red blood cells	promotes liver & kidney health	lowers cholesterol & blood pressure	stabilizes blood sugar
St. John's Wort	eases stress & depression	eases urinary tract infections	protects against radiation damage	beneficial for HIV & AIDS
Wheatgrass Juice	detoxifies the body	stabilizes blood sugar	anti-aging, anti-cancer	promotes liver & kidney health

~ Therapeutic Spices ~

Basil – (vitamins A, C & K, calcium, iron, magnesium, manganese, potassium)

Native to India and symbolizing love in Italy, basil is a nutrient-dense spice rich in antioxidants that help protect against many forms of cancer such as bladder, breast, colon, intestinal, lung, ovarian, pancreatic and prostate. A staple of Italian and Thai cuisine and honored by the ancient Greeks, this savory herb is a great source of beta carotene, and is effective for easing asthma, bronchitis, arthritis and inflammation. Basil is beneficial for lowering blood pressure and cholesterol, improving cardiovascular health, and protecting against diabetes by lowering blood sugar levels. It is effective for easing digestive disorders such as constipation and indigestion, and helps alleviate nausea as well. Basil improves skin disorders such as eczema and psoriasis, and helps protect cells and DNA from radiation damage. It is also an effective against bacterial, fungal and viral infections, and helps eliminate intestinal parasites.

Cayenne Pepper – (vitamins B1, B2, B3, B5, B6, C, E & K, calcium)

Cayenne pepper has been highly revered for thousands of years for its numerous life-extending health benefits. This red-hot chili pepper is rich in amino acids, and contains a powerful phytonutrient called *capsaicin* that protects DNA from carcinogens, inhibits tumor growth and destroys cancer cells. In addition to reducing the risk of most forms of cancer, cayenne pepper improves cardiovascular health, increases circulation, and helps protect against coronary heart disease. This spicy condiment is also effective for lowering blood pressure and cholesterol, controlling blood sugar levels, strengthening the immune system and alleviating arthritis and inflammation. Other benefits of this popular pepper include easing sinus infections, alleviating headaches and migraines, stimulating weight loss by increasing metabolism, improving digestion and helping to control flatulence. Often associated with cayenne pepper, paprika is generally a much milder spice that is dried and ground from sweet bell peppers. Chili powder is moderately spicy combination of cayenne pepper and paprika as well as cumin, garlic and oregano. * *Cayenne pepper should be avoided by those who have oral, stomach or esophageal cancer.*

Cilantro – (vitamin C, potassium)

Originally cultivated in the Mediterranean and the Middle East as far back as 5000 BC, cilantro is a fragrant spice that contains many therapeutic properties and is associated with immortality by the Chinese. Also referred to as "Chinese parsley," this nutrient-dense culinary herb is effective for improving many disorders such as arthritis, inflammation and muscle pain, normalizing blood sugar levels, lowering blood pressure and cholesterol and relieving migraine headaches. Rich in antioxidants, cilantro also helps protect against many forms of cancer, is effective at eliminating salmonella-based food poisoning, and is a great source of dietary fiber. Additionally, cilantro is beneficial for normalizing digestion and increasing appetite, and is commonly used as a mild sedative.

Cinnamon – (vitamins A, B1, B2, B3, C, calcium, iron, manganese, potassium, zinc)
Native to Sri Lanka and a favorite in China, cinnamon is an aromatic cooking spice that is loaded with health-promoting nutrients. It is effective for lowering blood pressure and cholesterol, inhibiting the proliferation of lymphoma and leukemia cancer cells, and controlling blood sugar levels. Cinnamon is beneficial for improving digestive disorders such as constipation, diarrhea, nausea, indigestion and irritable bowel syndrome, and is effective for stimulating weight loss. It also helps alleviate arthritis, inflammation, respiratory congestion and hoarseness, as well as increase brain function and improve memory. Furthermore, cinnamon provides powerful protection against yeast infections such as candida and thrush, and is effective against E. coli and other types of food poisoning.

Cumin – (vitamins A, B1, B2, B3, C, E & K, calcium, iron, magnesium, phosphorus, selenium, zinc)
Native to Egypt and belonging to the same plant family as dill and parsley, cumin is one of the main components of curry powder and has been used for centuries to spice up Indian and Middle Eastern cuisine. With a robust peppery/nutty flavor, cumin provides a long list of health benefits such as normalizing digestion, strengthening the immune system, and increasing respiratory health beneficial for those who suffer from asthma, bronchitis or the common cold. It contains anti-carcinogenic properties that inhibit tumor growth, and has shown promise in reducing the risk of breast and colon cancer. Cumin also contains iron beneficial for those who have anemia, and is essential for lactating mothers and women who are menstruating. Additionally, cumin increases cognitive function and memory, helps relieve insomnia, and improves skin ailments such as boils, insect bites and stings.

Dill – (vitamins A, B & C, calcium, iron, manganese, magnesium, phosphorus, potassium)
Dill is a tangy, flavorful herb that contains antibacterial properties, is rich in antioxidants, dietary fiber and mineral salts, and is a common spice used in salt-free diets. Once famous as a love potion ingredient and for its protection against witchcraft, dill has a calming effect on the stomach. It is effective for reducing a myriad of digestive disorders such as constipation, flatulence, indigestion, IBS and hemorrhoids, as well as vomiting and heartburn. The nutrients found in dill also lower the risk of

osteoporosis, help improve insomnia, alleviate arthritis and inflammation and help neutralize carcinogens from grilled foods and smoke. Furthermore, dill is beneficial for lowering blood pressure and cholesterol levels, and has been used to help alleviate menstrual discomforts.

Fennel – (vitamins B3, C, calcium, copper, folate, magnesium, manganese, phosphorus, potassium) Related to cilantro, dill and parsley, fennel is a popular Mediterranean spice that has a light, sweet, crunchy texture and has many health-promoting properties. It is an excellent source of antioxidants that help improve cardiovascular health, strengthen the immune system and reduce the risk of colon cancer. Fennel promotes proper kidney and liver function, is beneficial for those who have anemia, and helps alleviate arthritis and inflammation. It is also effective for easing asthma and bronchitis, and improving lung function. Fennel contains dietary fiber that lowers blood pressure and cholesterol levels, and helps normalizes digestive disorders such as constipation, diarrhea, heartburn, indigestion and irritable bowel syndrome. Additionally, it has been used for alleviating coughs, reducing fatigue, and has been known to help alleviate depression. For women, fennel is known to alleviate post-chemotherapy nausea and help control hormonal activity.

Garlic – (vitamins B1, B2, B3, B6, C, calcium, magnesium, manganese, selenium and zinc) Native to central Asia yet enjoyed throughout the world for over 6,000 years, garlic is one of the oldest and most highly regarded nutritional spices that has been used for improving a myriad of health disorders. Garlic was once so valuable that it was praised and used as currency by the ancient Egyptians. This highly flavorful bulb contains powerful, life-extending antioxidants that improve circulation, reduce the risk of heart attack and stroke, lower blood pressure and cholesterol levels and detoxify the blood. Garlic contains a sulfur compound called *allicin* which is effective for destroying cancer cells, inhibiting the growth of tumors, controlling blood sugar and supporting healthy liver function. Furthermore, garlic contains antibacterial and antiviral properties, and helps alleviate arthritis, asthma, bronchitis, strengthens the immune system and protects against colds, fevers and the flu.

Ginger – (vitamin A, B1, B2, B3, B6, C, calcium, magnesium, potassium, selenium, zinc) Originally cultivated in south Asia and India and well known for its powerful antioxidant properties, ginger has been used for thousands of years to successfully alleviate various digestive disorders such as motion sickness, nausea, vomiting and diarrhea. This sweet and pungent spice is also helpful for alleviating arthritis, inflammation, lowering cholesterol levels, controlling diabetes and protecting the liver. Ginger stimulates circulation and increases blood flow to the extremities, improves cardiovascular health, and reduces the risk of arteriosclerosis and atherosclerosis. It is also effective for relieving headaches, migraines, muscle cramps, menstrual discomforts and hot flashes. Ginger contains the same blood-thinning quality similar to aspirin that lowers the risk of heart attack or stroke, and protects against colds and the flu by strengthening the immune system. Additionally, it contains a phytonutrient called *zingibain* that is known to dissolve intestinal parasites and their eggs.

Mustard – (vitamin B3, calcium, iron, magnesium, phosphorus, protein, selenium, tryptophan, zinc)
Originally considered a medicinal plant and used for scorpion stings by the ancient Greeks, mustard is a savory spice that contains many phytonutrients and omega-3 fatty acids which help protect against the formation of cancer cells. It is beneficial for improving cardiovascular health, metabolism and reducing the risk of heart attacks associated with atherosclerosis. Providing an abundance of flavor with only a few calories, mustard helps alleviate arthritis and inflammation, lowers cholesterol levels and supports proper digestive function. It is also beneficial for strengthening the immune system, protecting against the common cold, and improving respiratory disorders such as asthma and bronchitis. Furthermore, mustard helps alleviate toothaches, and may reduce the frequency of migraine headaches.

Oregano – (vitamins A, C & K, calcium, iron, manganese)
Greek for "joy of the mountain," oregano is native to the hillsides of Greece and has been a favorite spice of Europe for thousands of years. It is a great source of fiber, omega-3 fatty acids and antioxidants that strengthen the immune system, reduce the risk of cancer and help lower blood pressure and cholesterol levels. This nutrient-dense herb helps alleviate a number of disorders such as indigestion, irritable bowel syndrome, diarrhea, flatulence and urinary tract infections. Oregano contains powerful antibiotic, antibacterial, antifungal and anti-parasitic properties, and for women is beneficial for eliminating yeast infections like candida and thrush. It is also helpful for relieving jaundice, reducing vomiting and is an effective cough suppressant. Drinking oregano tea steeped from the dried herb is another way to benefit from its health-promoting nutrients.

Parsley – (vitamin A, C, K, calcium, folate, iron, potassium)
Traced back the ancient Romans and native to the Mediterranean region of southern Europe, parsley is one of the most commonly used spices in the world. Rich in antioxidants and phytonutrients, parsley increases cardiovascular health, reduces the risk of many forms of cancer, and inhibits tumor growth in

the lungs by neutralizing carcinogens from smoke and environmental toxins. Used by Hippocrates himself for a variety of disorders, parsley is beneficial for strengthening the immune system, lowering blood pressure and cholesterol levels, and reducing plaque build-up in the arteries. Additionally, parsley helps to prevent water retention, and is rather effective for improving halitosis (bad breath).

Peppermint – (vitamin A, B2, C, calcium, folate, iron, magnesium, manganese, potassium)
Revered in Greek mythology for its sweet, minty aroma and a popular flavor for candy, gum, toothpaste and tea, peppermint is well known for soothing the stomach and improving gastrointestinal disorders like abdominal pain, bloating, constipation, diarrhea, flatulence and irritable bowel syndrome. This mouth-watering spice is a great source of omega-3 fatty acids, dietary fiber and various nutrients that improve cardiovascular health, and reduce the risk of cancer by inhibiting tumor growth. Peppermint is effective for easing headaches and migraines, reducing anxiety and tension, alleviating menstrual cramps and correcting insomnia. It contains *rosmarinic acid* which improves respiratory function and is beneficial for alleviating asthma and bronchitis. Furthermore, it is effective for alleviating allergies, quieting hiccups, reducing severe colds, and is effective for relieving mucus and nasal congestion. Peppermint is also known for preventing tooth decay, whitening teeth, protecting cells against carcinogens, and contains antibacterial properties that are beneficial for wounds and insect bites.

Rosemary – (calcium, iron)
Native to the Mediterranean and derived from its Latin name *ros marinus* meaning "dew of the sea," rosemary is one of the most widely respected herbs in the history of folklore, and is believed to have the ability to drive away illness, evil spirits and nightmares. An excellent addition to chicken, fish and a variety of soups, this pine-flavored spice is rich in dietary fiber and life-extending antioxidants that help reduce the risk of cancer and stimulate the immune system. Rosemary increases cognitive function, improves memory and concentration, and helps protect against senility and Alzheimer's disease by increasing blood flow to the brain. It promotes circulatory and nervous system health, reduces arthritis and inflammation, eases muscle pain and helps alleviate depression. Rosemary is also beneficial for reducing headaches, improving digestive disorders such as constipation, indigestion, irritable bowel syndrome and flatulence, relieving nausea and eliminating intestinal parasites.

Sage – (vitamins A, B & C, calcium, potassium)
Connected to folklore by its ability to increase wisdom, psychic powers and ward off evil, sage is a

savory, fragrant spice loaded with powerful antioxidants that has many nutritional benefits. Native to the Mediterranean region, sage is effective for inhibiting the growth of tumors and ulcers, and reducing the risk of cancer (especially lung). It is effective for increasing circulation, lowering cholesterol, alleviating arthritis and inflammation and protecting against atherosclerosis. Similar to rosemary, sage is beneficial for improving memory, concentration and brain function, and may help reduce the risk of Parkinson's disease. It promotes liver and kidney health, protects against gallstones, improves digestive disorders and helps control excessive sweating and hot flashes associated with menopause. Sage has been effectively used for alleviating night sweats associated with tuberculosis, and is also beneficial for asthma, bronchitis, colds, fevers and the flu. Additionally, sage eases inflammation of the mouth and gums, improves canker sores, and combined with chamomile tea is an effective gargle for sore throats.

Thyme – (vitamin K, calcium, iron, manganese)

Greek for "spirit", thyme is another nutrient-dense herb that for thousands of years has been utilized for both its flavor and health benefits. This savory spice is a great source of dietary fiber and contains powerful antioxidants that inhibit the growth of cancer cells. Thyme helps alleviate asthma, bronchitis, whooping cough and phlegm, improves respiratory function and soothes sore throats. An excellent complement to bean, egg and vegetables dishes, thyme is also helpful for lowering blood pressure and cholesterol, promoting liver health, alleviating arthritis and inflammation and contains strong antiseptic properties. Furthermore, thyme is known for relieving colds, fevers, headaches and easing flatulence.

Turmeric – (vitamins B1, B2, B3 & C, calcium, iron, potassium, zinc)

Originating in western India and utilized as flavoring, as a dye, and as medicine since 600 BC, turmeric is a powerful antioxidant that has been used to help reduce the risk of leukemia as well as many other forms of cancer including colon, breast, lung, ovarian, pancreatic, prostate, stomach and skin. Its active ingredient, *curcumin,* is beneficial for lowering cholesterol, alleviating arthritis, inflammation, asthma, bronchitis, relieving cystic fibrosis, and helps strengthen the cardiovascular system. Most commonly found in yellow curry and mustards, turmeric also improves liver health, strengthens the immune system and helps relieve the effects of food poisoning. This powerful super-spice increases blood circulation, improves intestinal flora, eliminates intestinal parasites and reduces the risk of developing polyps in the colon. Turmeric has also shown promise in breaking up the beta-amyloid plaques collected in the brain, which is considered one of the main causes of Alzheimer's disease. The elderly people of India rarely develop Alzheimer's disease, which is believed to be related to their regular consumption of turmeric.

Spices	Health Benefits			
Basil	alleviates asthma & bronchitis	lowers cholesterol & blood pressure	protects against diabetes	reduces arthritis & inflammation
Cayenne Pepper	strengthens the immune system	cardiovascular health	lowers cholesterol & blood pressure	reduces risk of atherosclerosis
Cilantro	reduces arthritis & inflammation	helps alleviate migraines	normalizes blood sugar levels	effective against food poisoning
Cinnamon	relieves nausea	improves respiratory health	eases digestive disorders	reduces arthritis & inflammation
Cumin	protects against colon cancer	eases digestive disorders	strengthens the immune system	improves respiratory health
Dill	eases digestive disorders	insomnia relief	reduces arthritis & inflammation	protects against osteoporosis
Fennel	promotes liver & kidney health	strengthens the immune system	lowers cholesterol & blood pressure	reduces arthritis & inflammation
Garlic	anti-cancer	detoxifies the blood	strengthens the immune system	lowers cholesterol & blood pressure
Ginger	relieves nausea	helps alleviate migraines	reduces arthritis & inflammation	eases symptoms of PMS
Mustard	cardiovascular health	reduces arthritis & inflammation	improves respiratory health	eases migraines
Oregano	lowers cholesterol & blood pressure	antibacterial & antiparasitic	anti-cancer & anti-aging	eases digestive disorders
Parsley	anti-cancer	lowers cholesterol & blood pressure	improves halitosis	cardiovascular health
Peppermint	eases digestive disorders	helps relieve insomnia	helps alleviate migraines	improves respiratory health
Rosemary	strengthens the immune system	Alzheimer's disease & senility	improves respiratory health	reduces arthritis & inflammation
Sage	anti-cancer	reduces arthritis & inflammation	eases respiratory infections	Alzheimer's disease & senility
Thyme	improves respiratory health	lowers cholesterol & blood pressure	effective against food poisoning	reduces colds & the flu
Turmeric	Alzheimer's disease & senility	anti-cancer	reduces arthritis & inflammation	lowers cholesterol & blood pressure

~ Holistic Herbs ~

Herbs are concentrated forms of plants, berries, roots and bark that provide vitamins, minerals and other nutrients which help strengthen the human body and promote vitality. They have been used by many ancient civilizations for a wide variety of therapeutic purposes, and have historically passed the test of time. Herbs were primarily helpful for restoring health and balance, seasoning foods and masking foul body odors. Because there was no refrigeration in the Middle Ages, herbs were used to preserve meat, and cover the taste of any foods that were not fresh. Native American tribes, like the Cherokee, Iroquois and Navajo, were well tenured in therapeutic herbal remedies and the nutritional benefits of their forest plants and shrubs. These tribes greatly understood and utilized their regional herbs for a myriad of different purposes like reducing the effects of fevers, colds, coughs, headaches, insect bites/stings, muscle aches, toothaches, digestive disorders, insomnia, syphilis and even certain blood disorders. Herbs are rich in phytonutrients that protect against premature aging, cancer, diabetes, mental decline and help strengthen the immune system. Certain herbs work best when taken alone, and some herbs are most productive when taken in conjunction with other herbs.

In the 21st century, herbs are becoming increasingly popular as a preventative health option. Herbal supplements do contain general health benefits, but everyone has different nutritional needs depending on their age, allergies, environment, genetics and overall health condition so the benefits are relative. Herbs that work well for one person may cause allergic reactions for another, which makes it imperative to know your allergies. During times of major injury, illness and/or surgery, nothing replaces the proper care of a knowledgeable doctor, and one should always consult their doctor before taking *any* new type of herbal health supplement – *especially pregnant women*!

Acerola – promotes liver health, reduces risk of atherosclerosis, alleviates diarrhea & constipation, relieves headaches, reduces fevers, hydrates the skin, beneficial for scurvy

Anise – improves digestive disorders, relieves mucus, phlegm & coughing, eases menopausal discomforts, alleviates nausea, reduces flatulence

Ashwagandha – stimulates the nervous system, promotes cardiovascular health, inhibits tumor growth, reduces arthritis & inflammation, strengthens the immune system, supports healthy adrenal gland function, helps relieve stress

Astragalus – strengthens the immune system, improves digestive disorders, increases energy & stamina, lowers risk of cancer & diabetes, supports healthy adrenal gland function, promotes lung health

Barberry – promotes liver & kidney health, relieves diarrhea & indigestion, fights bacterial infections of the skin, reduces fevers & sore throat, helps improve halitosis, decreases heart rate

Bayberry – improves circulation & varicose veins, promotes good vision, improves hypothyroidism, strengthens the immune system, helps reduce fevers and colds, sinus and respiratory relief, beneficial for ulcers, promotes eye health

Bilberry – promotes urinary tract health, reduces arthritis & inflammation, improves night vision, contains anti-aging properties, promotes skin health, helps regulate insulin levels, promotes eye health, eases stress & anxiety, contains antibacterial properties

Birch – reduces arthritis & inflammation, promotes urinary tract health, contains antiparasitic properties, natural pain reliever, improves boils & sores (topically)

Black Cohosh – lowers blood pressure & cholesterol, reduces arthritis & inflammation, promotes cardiovascular health, improves circulation, eases menstrual cramps, contains antiparasitic properties

Black Walnut – contains antiparasitic properties, improves digestive disorders, lowers blood pressure & cholesterol, beneficial for throat & mouth sores, helps alleviate bruising, protects against herpes, warts & fungal infections

Blessed Thistle – promotes liver health, strengthens the heart muscle, reduces arthritis & inflammation, improves circulation, cleanses the blood, contains antibacterial & antiviral properties

Blue Cohosh – eases menstrual discomforts, promotes a healthy uterus, reduces the risk of epilepsy, helps improve memory, relieves muscle spasms

Boldo – reduces arthritis & inflammation, promotes liver & pancreas health, reduces risk of gallstones, helps eliminate uric acid, effective diuretic & laxative

Boneset – relieves colds, fevers & the flu, reduces arthritis & inflammation, improves respiratory health, effective decongestant, diuretic & laxative, calming effects

Borage – promotes cardiovascular health, supports healthy adrenal gland function, reduces arthritis & inflammation, protects against eczema & psoriasis, helps reduce fevers, promotes healthy skin & nails

Boswellia – lowers blood pressure & cholesterol, reduces arthritis & inflammation, protects against obesity, helps alleviate diarrhea, beneficial for fibromyalgia and lower back pain, promotes liver health, contains antibacterial & antifungal properties

Buchu – protects against prostate disorders, promotes bladder & kidney health, reduces arthritis & inflammation, improves digestive disorders, beneficial for diabetes, effective as a diuretic

Burdock – promotes healthy liver & gallbladder function, cleanses the blood, improves skin disorders (boils), alleviates digestive disorders, strengthens the immune system, helps eliminate excess fluids, toxins & uric acid, eases menopausal discomforts, cleanses the blood, powerful anti-cancer properties

Butcher's Broom – reduces arthritis & inflammation, promotes bladder & kidney health, improves circulation & varicose veins, beneficial for Raynaud's disease and carpal tunnel syndrome, effective against hemorrhoids, protects against fluid retention & obesity

Calendula – beneficial for boils, rashes & sunburns, helps regulate menstrual cycles, reduces arthritis & inflammation, helps reduce fevers, contains antifungal properties

Cascara Sagrada – helps eliminate intestinal parasites, reduces the risk of gallstones, improves digestive disorders, promotes liver health, effective as a colon cleanse

Cat's Claw – lowers risk of cancer, tumors & ulcers, reduces arthritis & inflammation, strengthens the immune system, promotes gastrointestinal health, contains antiviral properties

Cedar – beneficial for bladder infections, strengthens the immune system, cleans the lymph glands, protects against genital warts, contains antifungal, antiviral & antiseptic properties

Chamomile – eases anxiety & stress, reduces arthritis & inflammation, improves digestive disorders, beneficial for colitis, helps alleviate headaches, fevers & menstrual cramps, improves insomnia

Chanca Piedra – promotes cardiovascular health, relieves gallstones & kidney stones, effective against STD's, reduces arthritis & inflammation, helps alleviate asthma & bronchitis, beneficial for sexually transmitted diseases (STD's), eases muscle spasms, helps alleviate colds and the flu, contains antibacterial & antiviral properties, effective diuretic

Chaparral – detoxifies the body, combats HIV & AIDS, anti-cancer properties, protects against skin disorders, natural pain reliever

Chaste Tree (agnus castus) – promotes gynecological health, regulates hormone levels, eases PMS and menopausal discomforts, supports the nervous system, helps relieve muscle cramps

Chickweed – improves circulation, helps alleviate bronchitis, coughs & colds, protects against skin disorders, effective against genital warts

Chicory – promotes liver & kidney health, improves urinary tract health, promotes spleen health, improves digestive disorders, detoxifies the body

Chuchuhuasi – inhibits tumor growth, promotes adrenal health, strengthens the immune system, helps alleviate back pain & muscle spasms, reduces arthritis & inflammation, beneficial for bronchitis, helps reduce fevers, alleviates diarrhea

Clove – helps eliminate intestinal parasites, eases toothache & mouth pain, improves digestive disorders, reduces arthritis & inflammation, contains antiseptic properties

Comfrey (topically) – promotes healing of wounds & burns, helps improve eczema, psoriasis & rashes, eases insect bites & stings, beneficial for bedsores, bruises & bunions, good for hemorrhoids

Corn Silk – promotes prostate health, eases carpal tunnel syndrome, supports liver & kidney health, promotes urinary tract health, protects against obesity, beneficial for edema, effective diuretic

Cramp Bark – helps relieve muscle spasms, reduces arthritis & inflammation, helps alleviate asthma & bronchitis, eases menstrual cramps, natural pain reliever

Damiana – improves infertility & impotence, reduces hot flashes from menopause, stimulates muscle contractions, controls hormone levels, natural aphrodisiac for women

Dandelion – promotes liver, kidney, pancreas & spleen health, lowers risk of breast cancer, eases menopausal discomforts, protects against skin disorders, cleanses the blood, reduces uric acid, lowers blood pressure & cholesterol, beneficial for anemia, improves constipation, effective diuretic

Dong Quai – eases PMS & menopausal discomforts, helps relieve muscle spasms, natural pain reliever, improves blood quality, effective diuretic & laxative

Elder – strengthens the immune system, improves respiratory health, relieves colds, congestion, fevers & the flu, reduces arthritis & inflammation, improves circulation, contains antiparasitic & antiviral properties, helps relieve constipation

Ephedra (Ma Huang) – stimulates the nervous system, increases energy & metabolism, helps improve respiratory health, effective appetite suppressant, helps alleviate allergies

Eucalyptus – improves respiratory health, helps relieve colds, sore throat & the flu, alleviates mucus, reduces arthritis & inflammation, helps relieve muscle pain

Eyebright – promotes good vision, reduces arthritis & inflammation, improves respiratory health, effective against allergies & hay fever, helps improve memory

Fenugreek – relieves coughs, fever & sore throat, beneficial for allergies, lowers blood pressure & cholesterol, eases headaches & migraines, improves respiratory health, alleviates asthma & sinus congestion, helps lower blood sugar levels, promotes eye health, effective laxative

Feverfew – helps reduce fevers, improves respiratory health, eases headaches & migraines, eases menstrual discomforts, reduces arthritis & inflammation, helps relieve nausea & vomiting, alleviates muscle spasms, tension & pain, beneficial for colitis

Gentian – improves digestive disorders, supports healthy gallbladder & liver function, protects against pancreatitis, improves circulation, helps reduce fevers & colds

Goldenseal – relieves colds, sore throat & the flu, alleviates bladder & digestive disorders, stimulates the nervous system, strengthens the immune system, promotes colon, liver, pancreas, spleen & prostate health, alleviates allergies, arthritis & inflammation, improves ulcers & mouth sores

Gotu Kola – helps improve memory, improves fatigue & depression, promotes healthy skin, improves circulation & cardiovascular health, beneficial for edema & varicose veins, helps eliminate kidney stones, supports healthy liver function, enhances wound healing, increases libido

Gravel Root – promotes urinary tract health, effective against kidney stones, helps alleviate fluid retention, promotes prostate health, effective diuretic

Guarana – powerful stimulant, increases endurance & mental alertness, promotes urinary tract health, eases headaches & migraines, effective intestinal cleanser

Hawthorn – lowers blood pressure & cholesterol, improves circulation, promotes cardiovascular health, beneficial for anemia, improves insomnia, helps relieve anxiety & stress

Hops – eases anxiety, nervousness & stress, helps alleviate insomnia, promotes cardiovascular health, beneficial for ulcers, natural pain reliever, alleviates toothaches

Horse Chestnut – promotes cardiovascular health, beneficial for varicose veins, protects against radiation damage, reduces arthritis & inflammation, eases muscle spasms & restless leg syndrome

Horsetail – promotes eyes, nose, ear & throat health, reduces arthritis & inflammation, strengthens bones, fingernails & hair, improves digestive disorders, promotes cardiovascular health

Hydrangea – protects against bladder & kidney infections, reduces arthritis & inflammation, promotes prostate health, beneficial for autoimmune disorders, protects against obesity

Hyssop – improves asthma, congestion & respiratory health, lowers blood pressure & cholesterol, reduces risk of epilepsy, beneficial for gout & obesity, improves circulation, helps reduce fevers

Irish Moss – eases indigestion, promotes urinary tract health, reduces risk of ulcers, reduces arthritis & inflammation, alleviates bronchitis

Jaborandi – reduces arthritis & inflammation, improves colds, fevers & the flu, beneficial for bronchitis, supports colon health, effective diuretic, used for baldness (topically)

Jatoba – helps improve respiratory health, alleviates asthma & bronchitis, reduces arthritis & inflammation, increases energy, promotes urinary tract health, beneficial for yeast infections, contains antibacterial & antifungal properties

Juniper – reduces arthritis & inflammation, promotes urinary tract health, cleanses the blood, protects against obesity, contains antiseptic & astringent properties

Kava Kava – helps relieve anxiety, stress & muscle spasms, improves digestive disorders, promotes urinary tract health, eases PMS & menopausal discomforts

Kudzu – helps alleviate alcohol cravings, lowers blood pressure & cholesterol, promotes gastrointestinal health, helps relieve headaches, good for colds & the flu

Lady's Mantle – promotes blood clotting, reduces arthritis & inflammation, helps regulate menstruation, eases cramps & muscle spasms, contains antiviral properties

Lavender – eases stress & anxiety, helps relieve headaches, improves insomnia & depression, beneficial for skin disorders (eczema & psoriasis)

Lemongrass – promotes gastrointestinal health, eases stress & anxiety, detoxifies intestinal tract, reduces skin disorders, improves circulation, eases flatulence, reduces uric acid, good for fevers

Licorice – contains antibacterial, antiviral and antiparasitic properties, beneficial for HIV & AIDS, improves circulatory health, reduces arthritis & inflammation, promotes liver & prostate health, relieves muscle spasms, eases PMS and menopausal discomforts, beneficial for allergies, asthma, bronchitis & emphysema, helps alleviate fatigue and depression

Maca – strengthens the immune system, eases PMS & menopausal discomforts, increases energy & strength, enhances the libido, helps improve impotence & infertility

Macela – promotes gastrointestinal health, lowers risk of Crohn's disease, beneficial for asthma & epilepsy, reduces muscle spasms, strengthens the immune system, eases PMS & menopausal discomforts, reduces arthritis & inflammation, good for colds & the flu

Marshmallow – promotes kidney & urinary tract health, eases diarrhea & Crohn's disease, improves respiratory health, alleviates fluid retention, promotes skin health, helps relieve headaches

Meadowsweet – improves diarrhea & digestive disorders, protects against ulcers, relieves cramps & muscle pain, reduces arthritis & inflammation, eases heartburn & nausea

Motherwort – eases menopausal & menstrual discomforts, helps relieve headaches, eases stress & anxiety, promotes cardiovascular health, beneficial for insomnia

Muira Puama – natural pain reliever, supports the nervous system, eases menopausal & menstrual discomforts, enhances libido & sexual function, detoxifies the body

Mullein – improves asthma & bronchitis, reduces arthritis & inflammation, alleviates congestion & sinus pressure, natural pain reliever, effective against allergies & hay fever, effective laxative

Myrrh – reduces cold sores & canker sores, improves digestive disorders, strengthens the immune system, helps alleviate asthma & bronchitis, beneficial for skin disorders (abscesses, boils & wounds), improves gingivitis & halitosis, good for colds, fevers & the flu

Nettle – promotes kidney & urinary tract health, lowers risk of BPH (enlarged prostate), helps improve respiratory health, helps reduce colds, congestion & fevers, beneficial for anemia, helps alleviate allergies & hay fever, reduces arthritis & inflammation, effective diuretic

Oat Straw – stimulates the nervous system, beneficial for varicose veins, lowers blood pressure & cholesterol, protects against skin disorders (shingles), improves insomnia, eases anxiety & stress

Olive Leaf – contains antibacterial, antifungal, antiviral, antiparasitic properties, helps lower blood pressure, reduces fatigue, good for colds, fevers & the flu, strengthens the immune system, reduces arthritis & inflammation, alleviates diarrhea, beneficial for skin disorders (eczema & psoriasis)

Oregon Grape – reduces arthritis & inflammation, helps improve liver disorders (jaundice, cirrhosis & hepatitis), beneficial for skin disorders (psoriasis), promotes urinary tract health, cleanses the blood

Passionflower – eases anxiety, stress & nausea, lowers blood pressure, alleviates asthma & respiratory disorders, improves digestive disorders, beneficial for alcoholism

Pau d'Arco – promotes cardiovascular & respiratory health, inhibits growth of tumors & ulcers, strengthens the immune system, reduces arthritis & inflammation, promotes skin health, contains antibacterial, antifungal & antiviral properties, beneficial for HIV & AIDS, helps eliminate intestinal parasites, reduces yeast infections, alleviates hemorrhoids, good for colds, fevers & the flu

Plantain – promotes urinary tract health, beneficial for tuberculosis, relieves heartburn & hemorrhoids, improves respiratory health, beneficial for sores & wounds, insect bites, bee stings & poison ivy

Pleurisy Root – reduces arthritis & inflammation, alleviates asthma & bronchitis, eases menopausal & menstrual disorders, alleviates diarrhea, beneficial for coughs, fevers, pneumonia & the flu

Primrose – lowers blood pressure & cholesterol, eases PMS & menopausal discomforts, beneficial for skin disorders (eczema & rosacea), protects against osteoporosis, reduces arthritis & inflammation, beneficial for impotence, infertility, senility and lupus

Puncture Vine – lowers blood pressure & cholesterol, lowers the risk of arteriosclerosis & atherosclerosis, promotes liver, kidney & urinary tract health, stimulates the immune system, enhances muscle building & endurance, stimulates the libido, eases menopausal symptoms, mild diuretic

Pygeum – promotes prostate health, alleviates congestion, reduces arthritis & inflammation, promotes urinary tract health, alleviates painful urination

Red Clover – cleanses the blood, lowers blood pressure & cholesterol, protects against diabetes, beneficial for HIV & AIDS, improves respiratory health, strengthens the immune system, beneficial for liver & kidney disorders, eases menopausal discomforts, alleviates digestive disorders

Rose – beneficial for bladder infections, improves respiratory health, reduces risk of arteriosclerosis, helps alleviate diarrhea, contains antiseptic & antiviral properties

Sangre de Grado – alleviates bacterial, fungal & viral infections (herpes, yeast infections), inhibits the growth of tumors, beneficial for skin disorders (ulcers, psoriasis), enhances wound healing, improves respiratory health, relieves colds, sore throat & the flu

Sarsaparilla – reduces risk of radiation damage, promotes liver health, alleviates arthritis & gout, helps regulate hormones, nervous system health, eases menopausal discomforts, improves infertility/impotence

Skullcap – promotes nervous system health, alleviates cramps & muscle spasms, improves circulation & digestion, eases stress & anxiety, protects against cardiovascular disease, improves insomnia & fatigue, effective hangover remedy

Slippery Elm – promotes kidney & urinary tract health, beneficial for Crohn's disease, colitis & diverticulitis, relieves colds, sore throat & the flu, eases heartburn, ulcers & indigestion, helps alleviate constipation, diarrhea & hemorrhoids

Squaw Vine – promotes healthy nervous system, helps relieve menstrual cramps, natural sedative properties, strengthens the uterus & helps prevent miscarriages, beneficial at childbirth

Tea Tree – promotes health skin, improves respiratory health, beneficial for measles & chicken pox, strengthens the immune system, contains antibacterial, antifungal & antiviral properties

Uva Ursi – strengthens the heart & spleen, protects against bladder & kidney infections, beneficial for kidney stones, promotes pancreas & prostate health, protects against diabetes

Valerian – improves circulation, lowers blood pressure & cholesterol, promotes healthy nervous system, eases irritable bowel syndrome, natural sedative & pain reliever, eases stress & anxiety, improves insomnia, relieves menstrual cramps

Vervain – promotes nervous system & respiratory health, supports liver & gallbladder health, alleviates menstrual discomforts, eases anxiety & stress, relieves colds, fever & the flu, helps alleviate depression

White Oak – beneficial for gallstones & kidney stones, relieves colds, fever & the flu, reduces varicose veins, contains antiseptic properties, beneficial for skin disorders (burns, insect stings, poison ivy, wounds), helps alleviate diarrhea & hemorrhoids

White Willow – natural pain reliever, reduces arthritis & inflammation, alleviates indigestion & heartburn, relieves colds, fever & the flu, eases menstrual cramps

Wild Cherry – promotes lung, pancreas & spleen health, alleviates asthma & bronchitis, eases diarrhea & digestive disorders, relieves coughs & colds, mild sedative

Wintergreen – improves respiratory health, reduces arthritis & inflammation, natural pain reliever, improves circulation, alleviates constipation

Wood Betony – relieves heartburn & indigestion, cleanses the blood, promotes cardiovascular & respiratory health, contains antiparasitic properties, eases headaches, anxiety & stress

Wormwood – contains antiparasitic properties, supports liver & gallbladder health, helps reduce fevers, eases headaches & migraines, beneficial for skin disorders (insect stings, ulcers, wounds)

Yellow Dock – promotes healthy liver function, cleanses the blood & lymphatic system, improves respiratory health, protects against anemia, inhibits the growth of tumors, contains antiparasitic properties, beneficial for skin disorders (eczema, psoriasis, hives & rashes)

Yerba Buena – powerful pain relief, eases flatulence & indigestion, helps relieve headaches, relieves muscle & joint pain, beneficial for halitosis

Yerba Mate – promotes nervous system health, contains anti-aging properties, cleanses the blood, eases heartburn & indigestion, beneficial for allergies

Yohimbe – beneficial for erectile dysfunction, natural aphrodisiac, relieves colds, fevers & the flu, improves circulation, may increase testosterone levels

Yucca – cleanses the blood, protects against osteoporosis, reduces arthritis & inflammation, eases headaches & migraines, beneficial for gonorrhea

Herbs	Health Benefits			
Acerola	promotes liver health	reduces risk of atherosclerosis	beneficial for scurvy	alleviates constipation
Anise	eases digestive disorders	relieves mucus, phlegm, coughing	eases menopausal discomforts	alleviates nausea & flatulence
Ashwagandha	stimulates the nervous system	cardiovascular health	helps relieve stress	reduces arthritis & inflammation
Astragalus	eases digestive disorders	increases energy & stamina	lowers risk of cancer & diabetes	improves respiratory health
Barberry	alleviates diarrhea & indigestion	promotes liver & kidney health	beneficial for skin disorders/infections	eases fevers & sore throat
Bayberry	circulation & varicose veins	helps reduce fever and colds	promotes good vision	improves hypothyroidism
Bilberry	promotes urinary tract health	macular degeneration	eases anxiety & stress	reduces arthritis & inflammation
Birch	reduces arthritis & inflammation	improves boils & sores (topically)	promotes urinary tract health	helps eliminate intestinal parasites
Black Cohosh	lowers cholesterol & blood pressure	helps eliminate intestinal parasites	cardiovascular health	eases menopausal symptoms
Black Walnut	eases digestive disorders	protests against herpes & warts	helps eliminate intestinal parasites	eases throat & mouth sores
Blessed Thistle	strengthens heart muscle	cirrhosis & hepatitis	reduces arthritis & inflammation	improves circulation
Blue Cohosh	promotes healthy uterus	eases menstrual discomforts	helps improve memory	reduces risk of epilepsy
Boldo	reduces arthritis & inflammation	reduces risk of pancreatic cancer	reduces risk of gallstones	improves jaundice & liver disorders
Boneset	relieves colds, fever & the flu	effective diuretic & laxative	improves respiratory health	reduces arthritis & inflammation
Borage	cardiovascular health	eczema & psoriasis	supports healthy adrenal gland	helps reduce fevers

Herbs	Health Benefits			
Boswellia	lowers cholesterol & blood pressure	reduces arthritis & inflammation	antibacterial & antifungal	protects against obesity
Buchu	promotes prostate health	improves digestive disorders	promotes bladder & kidney health	reduces arthritis & inflammation
Burdock	cleanses the blood	gallbladder & liver function	beneficial for skin disorders	digestive disorders
Butcher's Broom	reduces arthritis & inflammation	hemorrhoids, fluid retention & obesity	circulation & varicose veins	promotes bladder & kidney health
Calendula	helps regulate menstrual cycles	reduces arthritis & inflammation	helps reduce fevers	beneficial for boils sunburns & rashes
Cascara Sagrada	helps eliminate intestinal parasites	reduces risk of gallstones	improves digestive disorders	promotes liver health
Cat's Claw	reduces arthritis & inflammation	good for cancer, tumors & ulcers	promotes intestinal tract health	strengthens the immune system
Cedar	antiviral, antifungal	cleans the lymph glands	strengthens the immune system	beneficial for bladder infections
Chamomile	eases anxiety & stress	reduces arthritis & inflammation	improves digestive disorders	eases colitis & menstrual cramps
Chanca Piedra	antibacterial & antiviral	eases asthma & bronchitis	relieves gallstones & kidney stones	effective against STD's
Chaparral	detoxifies the body	combats HIV & AIDS	beneficial for skin disorders	natural pain reliever
Chaste Tree	eases menopausal & PMS symptoms	controls hormone levels	gastrointestinal health	supports the nervous system
Chickweed	improves circulation	alleviates bronchitis	beneficial for skin disorders	helps alleviate coughs & colds
Chicory	promotes liver & kidney health	improves urinary tract health	promotes spleen health	improves digestive disorders
Chuchuhuasi	reduces arthritis & inflammation	promotes adrenal health	eases back pain & muscle spasms	inhibits tumor growth

Herbs	Health Benefits			
Clove	helps eliminate intestinal parasites	improves digestive disorders	eases toothache & mouth pain	reduces arthritis & inflammation
Comfrey	promotes healing of wounds & burns	beneficial for hemorrhoids	good for eczema, psoriasis & rashes	alleviates insect bites & stings
Corn Silk	promotes prostate health	supports liver & kidney health	eases carpal tunnel syndrome	promotes urinary tract health
Cramp Bark	helps relieve muscle spasms	eases asthma & bronchitis	reduces arthritis & inflammation	eases menstrual cramps
Damiana	stimulates muscle contractions	improves infertility & impotence	reduces hot flashes from menopause	controls hormone levels
Dandelion	promotes liver health	lowers cholesterol & blood pressure	promotes kidney & spleen health	beneficial for skin disorders
Dong Quai	improves blood quality	natural pain reliever	eases menopausal discomforts	helps relieve muscle spasms
Elder	helps eliminate intestinal parasites	reduces arthritis & inflammation	improves respiratory health	relieves colds, fever & the flu
Ephedra (ma huang)	stimulates nervous system	improves respiratory health	increases energy & metabolism	appetite suppressant
Eucalyptus	improves respiratory health	colds, sore throat & the flu	reduces arthritis & inflammation	helps relieve muscle pain
Eyebright	promotes good vision	helps improve memory	eases allergies & hay fever	reduces arthritis & inflammation
Fenugreek	relieves coughs, fever & sore throat	alleviates asthma & sinus congestion	lowers cholesterol & blood pressure	eases headaches & migraines
Feverfew	helps reduce fevers	eases headaches & migraines	reduces arthritis & inflammation	improves respiratory health
Gentian	improves digestive disorders	beneficial for colds & fevers	gallbladder & liver health	protects against pancreatitis
Goldenseal	relieves colds, sore throat & the flu	reduces arthritis & inflammation	strengthens the immune system	liver, pancreas, prostate & spleen

Herbs	Health Benefits			
Gotu Kola	helps improve memory	improves fatigue & depression	circulation & varicose veins	helps eliminate kidney stones
Gravel Root	promotes urinary tract health	effective diuretic	beneficial for kidney stones	promotes prostate health
Guarana	powerful stimulant	endurance & mental alertness	promotes urinary tract health	eases headaches & migraines
Hawthorn	lowers cholesterol & blood pressure	cardiovascular health	improves circulation	eases anxiety & stress
Hops	eases anxiety & stress	improves insomnia	cardiovascular health	beneficial for ulcers
Horse Chestnut	cardiovascular health	beneficial for varicose veins	alleviates muscle spasms	reduces arthritis & inflammation
Horsetail	eyes, nose, ear & throat health	reduces arthritis & inflammation	strengthens bones, fingernails & hair	improves digestive disorders
Hydrangea	promotes bladder & kidney health	protects against obesity	reduces arthritis & inflammation	promotes prostate health
Hyssop	improves respiratory health	lowers cholesterol & blood pressure	improves circulation	protects against obesity
Irish Moss	reduces ulcers & digestive disorders	reduces arthritis & inflammation	promotes urinary tract health	alleviates bronchitis
Jaborandi	reduces arthritis & inflammation	beneficial for bronchitis	improves colds, fevers & the flu	supports colon health
Jatoba	improves respiratory health	antibacterial & antifungal	reduces arthritis & inflammation	promotes urinary tract health
Juniper	reduces arthritis & inflammation	promotes urinary tract health	cleanses the blood	protects against obesity
Kava Kava	eases anxiety & stress	improves digestive disorders	promotes urinary tract health	eases menopausal discomforts
Kudzu	helps alleviate alcohol cravings	beneficial for colds & the flu	lowers cholesterol & blood pressure	gastrointestinal health

Herbs	Health Benefits			
Lady's Mantle	reduces arthritis & inflammation	promotes blood clotting	eases cramps & muscle spasms	helps regulate menstruation
Lavender	eases anxiety & stress	improves insomnia	beneficial for skin disorders	helps relieve headaches
Lemongrass	detoxifies intestinal tract	eases anxiety & stress	reduces uric acid (improves gout)	improves circulation
Licorice	helps eliminate intestinal parasites	beneficial for HIV & AIDS	promotes liver & prostate health	circulatory & respiratory health
Maca	strengthens the immune system	eases menopausal discomforts	increases energy & strength	infertility & impotence
Macela	eases menopausal discomforts	protects against Crohn's disease	strengthens the immune system	beneficial for asthma & epilepsy
Marshmallow	urinary tract & kidney & health	eases diarrhea & Crohn's disease	helps alleviate fluid retention	beneficial for skin disorders
Meadowsweet	arthritis, cramps, muscle pain	protects against ulcers	improves digestive disorders	eases heartburn & nausea
Motherwort	eases menopausal disorders	helps relieve headaches	cardiovascular health	eases anxiety & stress
Muira Puama	natural pain reliever	eases menopausal disorders	supports the nervous system	enhances libido & sexual function
Mullein	eases asthma & bronchitis	reduces arthritis & inflammation	alleviates allergies & sinus pressure	natural pain reliever
Myrrh	reduces cold sores & canker sores	improves digestive disorders	good for colds, fevers & the flu	gingivitis & halitosis
Nettle	urinary tract & kidney & health	beneficial for colds & fevers	improves respiratory health	lowers risk of enlarged prostate
Oat Straw	stimulates the nervous system	beneficial for varicose veins	lowers cholesterol & blood pressure	beneficial for skin disorders
Olive Leaf	antibacterial & antiviral	lowers cholesterol & blood pressure	good for colds, fevers & the flu	eczema & psoriasis

Herbs	Health Benefits			
Oregon Grape	jaundice, cirrhosis & hepatitis	cleanses the blood	beneficial for skin disorders	reduces arthritis & inflammation
Passionflower	eases anxiety, stress & nausea	beneficial for alcoholism	eases respiratory disorders	lowers blood pressure
Pau d'Arco	antibacterial, antiviral	cardiovascular health	inhibits growth of tumors & ulcers	lupus & tuberculosis
Plantain	beneficial for tuberculosis	promotes urinary tract health	relieves heartburn & hemorrhoids	insect bites, poison ivy
Pleurisy Root	reduces arthritis & inflammation	eases asthma & bronchitis	eases menopausal disorders	relieves coughs, fevers, the flu
Primrose	lowers cholesterol & blood pressure	eases menopausal discomforts	infertility & impotence	protects against osteoporosis
Puncture Vine	lowers cholesterol & blood pressure	arteriosclerosis & atherosclerosis	liver, kidneys & urinary tract	eases menopausal disorders
Pygeum	alleviates congestion	promotes prostate health	reduces arthritis & inflammation	urinary tract health
Red Clover	cleanses the blood	beneficial for HIV & AIDS	eases menopausal discomforts	relieves IBS, indigestion
Rose	beneficial for bladder infections	reduces risk of arteriosclerosis	helps alleviate diarrhea	respiratory health
Sangre de Grado	antibacterial, antiviral	colds, sore throat & the flu	beneficial for skin disorders	inhibits growth of tumors/ulcers
Sarsaparilla	reduces risk of radiation damage	promotes liver & hormone health	alleviates arthritis & gout	infertility & impotence
Skullcap	promotes nervous system health	circulation & digestion	eases cramps & muscle spasms	hangover remedy
Slippery Elm	urinary tract & kidney health	eases constipation & hemorrhoids	eases heartburn & indigestion	Crohn's disease, diverticulitis
Squaw Vine	promotes healthy nervous system	helps relieve menstrual cramps	beneficial at childbirth	strengthens the uterus

Herbs	Health Benefits			
Tea Tree	promotes healthy skin (topically)	improves respiratory health	alleviates measles & chicken pox	antibacterial, antiviral
Uva Ursi	strengthens the heart & spleen	eases bladder & kidney infections	promotes prostate health	protects against diabetes
Valerian	improves circulation	eases menstrual cramps	promotes healthy nervous system	lowers cholesterol & blood pressure
Vervain	nervous system & respiratory health	eases menstrual discomforts	gallbladder & liver function	relieves colds, fever & the flu
White Oak	reduces gallstones & kidney stones	eases diarrhea & hemorrhoids	burns, insect stings, poison ivy	beneficial for varicose veins
White Willow	natural pain reliever	eases indigestion & heartburn	relieves colds, fever & the flu	eases menstrual cramps
Wild Cherry	eases asthma & bronchitis	relieves coughs & colds	lung, pancreas & spleen health	eases diarrhea & digestive disorders
Wintergreen	improves respiratory health	reduces arthritis & inflammation	alleviates constipation	improves circulation
Wood Betony	cardiovascular & respiratory health	relieves heartburn & indigestion	eases headaches, anxiety & stress	helps eliminate intestinal parasites
Wormwood	helps eliminate intestinal parasites	gallbladder & liver function	beneficial for skin disorders	eases headaches & migraines
Yellow Dock	protects against anemia	promotes healthy liver function	improves respiratory health	hives, rashes, eczema, psoriasis
Yerba Buena	powerful pain relief	eases flatulence & indigestion	eases headaches & joint pain	beneficial for halitosis
Yerba Mate	eases heartburn & indigestion	cleanses the blood	promotes nervous system health	beneficial for allergies
Yohimbe	erectile dysfunction	natural aphrodisiac	relieves colds, fevers & the flu	improves circulation
Yucca	cleanses the blood	protects against osteoporosis	reduces arthritis & inflammation	eases headaches & migraines

~ Caution When Taking Herbs & Supplements ~

It is vital to understand the possible benefits and side effects of foods and nutrients. Listed below are common health conditions and specific foods, herbs & supplements that should ***NEVER*** be combined. Know your allergies, and always consult your physician before taking any new supplement, herb or consuming unfamiliar foods. (Example: if you have allergies to shellfish - do not take glucosamine)

AVOID THESE FOODS, HERBS & SUPPLEMENTS if you have the following conditions:

Alkalosis – *avoid* aloe vera juice

Allergies – *avoid* chamomile, echinacea

Allergies to shellfish – *avoid* glucosamine

Anxiety – *avoid* yohimbe

Arthritis – *avoid* echinacea

Asthma – *avoid* chondroitin, dairy, St. John's wort

Autoimmune disorders – *avoid* echinacea

Cardiovascular disease – *avoid* licorice

Celiac disease – *avoid* barley, bulgur, couscous, durum, echinacea, kamut, oats, rye, spelt and wheat

Cirrhosis – *avoid* black cohosh, chaparral, comfrey, vanadium, yohimbe

Crohn's disease – *avoid* echinacea, Irish moss

Colitis – *avoid* echinacea

Dementia – *avoid* St. John's wort

Diabetes – *avoid* dong quai, echinacea, ephedra, glucosamine, licorice

Diarrhea – *avoid* aloe vera juice, brewer's yeast

Epilepsy (*seizures*) – *avoid* chondroitin, eucalyptus, fennel, ginkgo biloba, rosemary, sage, St. John's wort

Fever – *avoid* astragalus

Gallstones – *avoid* dandelion

Glaucoma – *avoid* licorice

Gout – *avoid* brewer's yeast

Hemophilia – *avoid* garlic, ginger, ginkgo biloba, ginseng, horse chestnut, meadowsweet, onions, turmeric, white willow

Hepatitis – *avoid* black cohosh, chaparral, comfrey, echinacea, vanadium, yohimbe

High blood pressure (*hypertension*) – *avoid* brewer's yeast, ephedra, ginger, ginseng, guarana, licorice, motherwort, rosemary, saw palmetto, St. John's wort, yohimbe

High cholesterol – *avoid* saw palmetto

Hyperthyroidism – *avoid* kelp

Hypothyroidism – *avoid* kale

Hypoglycemia (*low blood sugar*) – *avoid* cordyceps, ginseng

Inflammation – *avoid* echinacea

Intestinal disorders (except constipation) – *avoid* brewer's yeast

Insomnia – *avoid* ginseng

Kidney disease – *avoid* juniper, vanadium

Lupus – *avoid* alfalfa sprouts, caffeine, cayenne pepper, citrus fruits, dairy, echinacea, eggs, fluorescent lighting, nightshade vegetables (bell peppers, eggplant, tomatoes, white potatoes), paprika, red meat, sodium

Melanoma – *avoid* cordyceps, fennel, garlic, licorice

Multiple Sclerosis – *avoid* echinacea

Parkinson's disease – *avoid* graviola

Poor iron absorption – *avoid* bilberry, burdock, damiana, juniper, lady's mantle, peppermint, sage, vervain

Prostate cancer – *avoid* excessive dairy

Viral infections (*AIDS/HIV, chicken pox, herpes, HPV, influenza, warts*) – *avoid* meadowsweet

Part Three

Personal Health and Nutrition

~ Okinawa Diet Food Pyramid ~

The people of Okinawa Japan have the longest life expectancy in the world. Wonder why? In addition to genetics and a peaceful, slower-paced lifestyle, much of Okinawan longevity is attributed to their local diet. The Okinawan diet consists of nutrient-dense, low calorie, low-fat foods including fresh fish, organic vegetables, whole grains, soy foods and legumes. It also advocates the importance of calcium intake, complex carbohydrates, omega 3's and limiting the consumption of red meat. The Okinawa diet suggests eating slowly and thoroughly chewing food, eating small portions, stopping before you are full and consuming a wide variety of nutrients for maximizing nutritional intake. The Okinawa culture also emphasizes the importance of daily exercise, strength training and aerobic activities including tai chi and yoga, as well as meditation, staying relaxed and thinking positive.

Bradley Willcox, M.D., M.S., an international expert on healthy aging, a Physician Investigator in Geriatrics and Co-Principle Investigator of the Okinawan Centenarian Study, along with Craig Willcox, Ph.D., M.H.Sc., anthropology and epidemiology expert and Professor of Gerontology and International Public Health & Welfare, and Makoto Suzuki, M.D., Ph.D., cardiologist, geriatrician, Director at the Okinawa Research Center for Longevity Science and Principle Investigator of the Okinawan Centenarian Study, co-authored the vitally informative book titled *The Okinawan Diet Plan – Get Leaner, Live Longer and Never Feel Hungry*. It provides three various dietary guideline options including the Eastern/Okinawan, East-West Fusion and Western diet plans, and also addresses the vegetarian diet for maintaining proper weight and health. The main focus of the Okinawa diet plan is on calorie density (CD) which is the number of calories per 1 gram. Foods are categorized according to their caloric density rates of "Featherweights" (0 – 0.7 CD), "Lightweights" (0.8 – 1.5 CD), "Middleweights" (1.6 – 3.0 CD) foods which should be consumed in moderation and "Heavyweights" (3.1 – 9.0 CD) of which consumption should be minimal. Caloric density can be calculated by dividing the serving size in grams into the calories per servings. For example, peanut butter has 190 calories per serving and a serving size is 32 grams which equals 5.9 CD (190 / 32 = 5.9375) and should be consumed in moderation. Low-fat cottage cheese has 90 calories per serving and a serving size is 113 grams which equals .8 CD (90 / 113 = 0.7964) and may be consumed more frequently.

These highly accredited and well respected doctors also co-authored another important book titled *The Okinawa Program – How the World's Longest-lived People Achieve Everlasting Health-and how you can too.* Through extensive research they have created the "Okinawa Diet Food Pyramid," displayed on the following page, which illustrates the traditional diet of the Okinawan people. For more information, please visit www.okinawa-diet.com.

The Okinawa Diet Food Pyramid

A Guide to Daily Food Choices

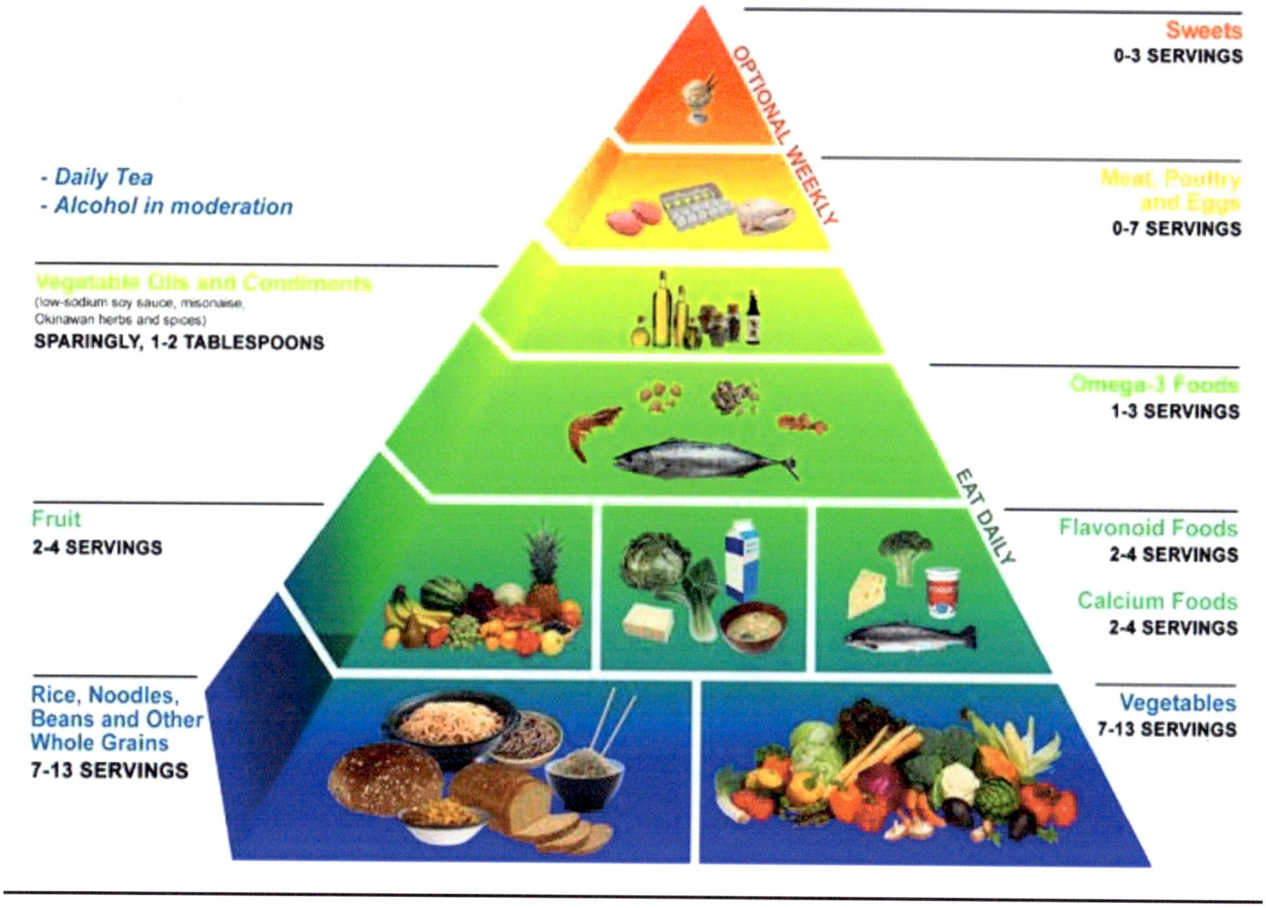

~ Asian & Mediterranean Food Pyramids ~

Various organizations have created their own versions of food guide pyramids including researchers from Harvard's School of Public Health, Cornell-China-Oxford Project on Nutritional Health and Environment, the World Health Organization (WHO) and the United States Department of Agriculture (USDA). The Oldways Preservation & Exchange Trust, in conjunction with those organizations listed above, has created many of the popular food guide pyramids of today. These informative food pyramids illustrate the different food groupings among various cultures and display their unique, traditional recommendations. The following pages showcase the most highly revered and widely studied Asian and Mediterranean Diet Pyramids. For a complete list of all food pyramids from the Oldways Preservation & Exchange Trust, please visit *www.oldwayspt.org*.

Asian Diet Pyramid: The people of Asia are among those with the longest life expectancy due to low rates of chronic degenerative diseases. The Asian Diet Pyramid is based on the dietary traditions of a broad range of countries including Bangladesh, Cambodia, China, India, Indonesian, Japan, Laos, Malaysia, Mongolia, Myanmar (Burma), Nepal, North Korea, South Korea, Malaysia, Philippines, Singapore, Taiwan, Thailand and Vietnam. Although every Asian country has unique foods, flavors and culinary traditions based on their particular region, rice is the one common staple food among all of these countries. The Asian diet is also rich in plant foods including fruits, vegetables, beans, nuts, grains, onions and vegetable oil. Other foods include fish, poultry and eggs, yet the consumption of dairy, red meat and sweets are limited.

Mediterranean Diet Pyramid: The people of the Mediterranean region also enjoy a long life expectancy and have much lower rates of chronic degenerative diseases than people of the West. The Mediterranean Diet Pyramid is based on the traditional diet of Crete, Greece and southern Italy. Their diet consists mainly of fruits, vegetables, beans, breads, grains, nuts/seeds, potatoes and olive oil. Dairy foods like cheese and yogurt are consumed in small amounts on a daily basis. Fresh fruit and honey are limited to a few times a week. Moderate amounts of fish and poultry are consumed twice a week and lean red meat is limited to a couple times per month. Red wine is also on the menu, but is consumed in moderation only and usually with meals. The Mediterranean diet emphasizes the importance of organic, locally-grown plant foods to maximize nutritional intake. Epidemiological research suggests this is a major factor in the longevity of the Mediterranean culture.

The Traditional Healthy Asian Diet Pyramid

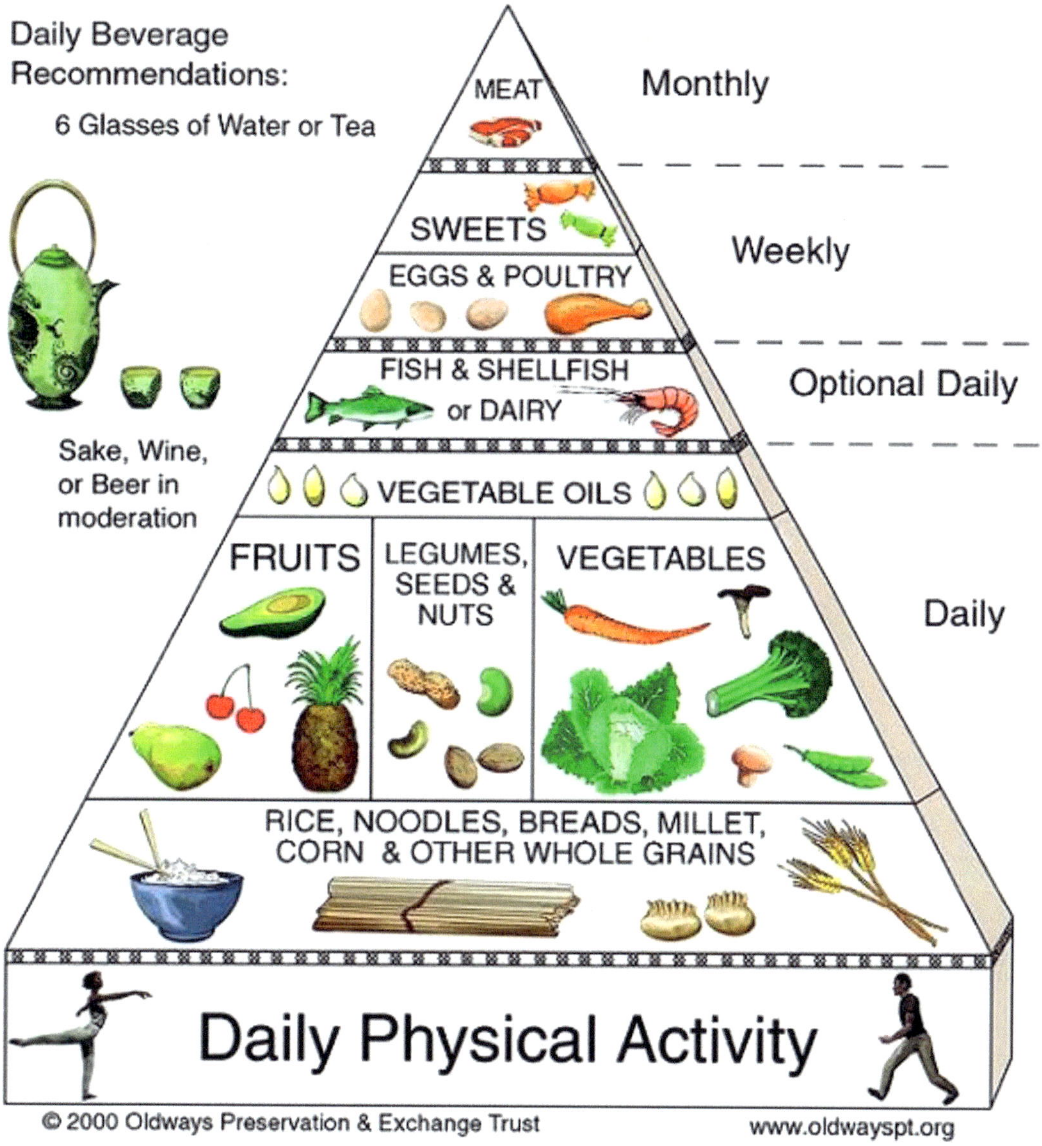

The Traditional Healthy Mediterranean Diet Pyramid

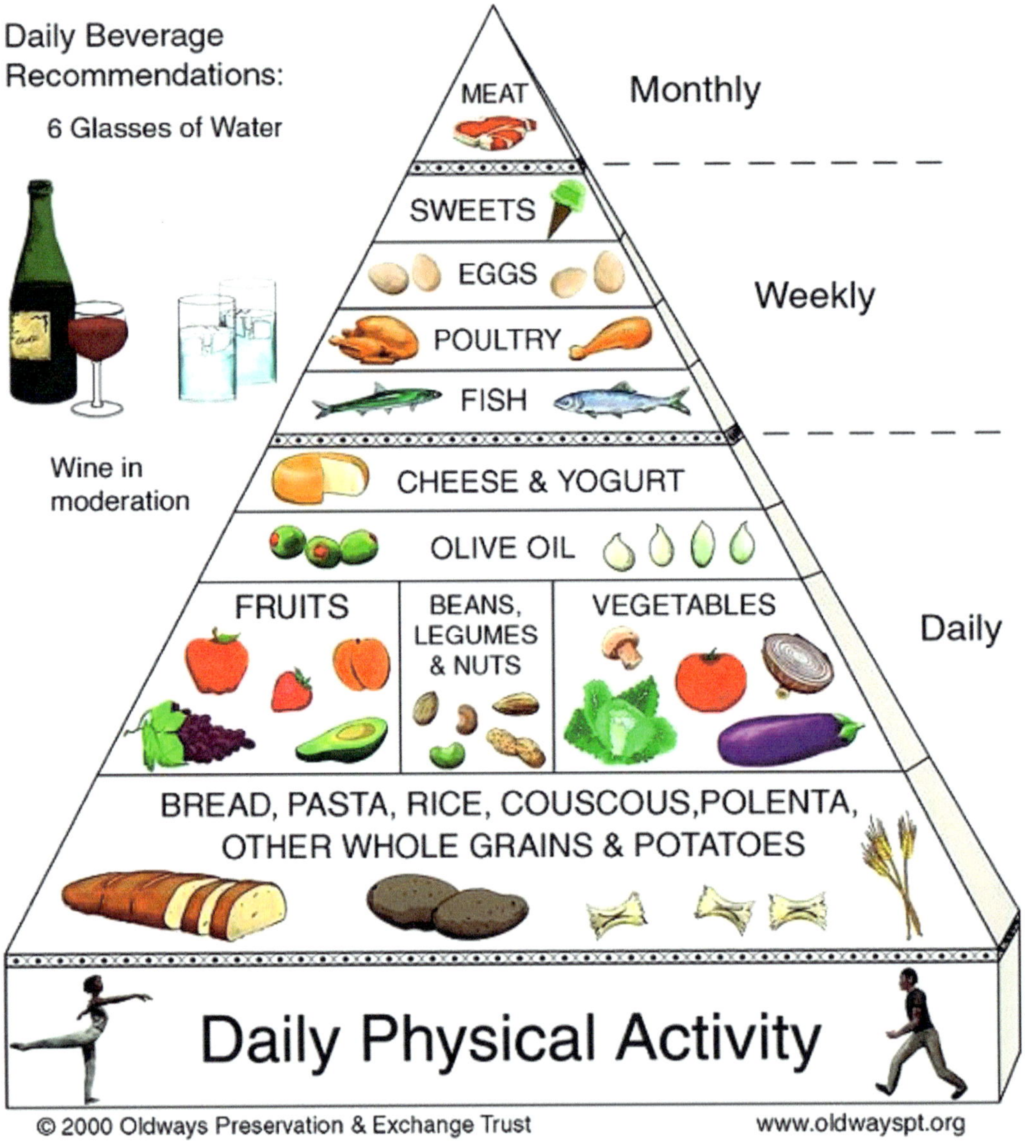

~ Optimal Health Food Pyramid ~

Dr. Michael T. Murray, N.D., consultant, educator, lecturer and researcher to the healthy food industry, along with cofounder of Bastyr University Joseph Pizzorno, N.D. and health writer and medical editor Lara Pizzorno, M.A., L.M.T., co-authored the exceptionally informative book titled *The Encyclopedia of Healing Foods*. They are among the most revered experts in the field of nutrition and natural medicine addressing important issues and inspiring us to make healthier food choices. Their book explains the nutritional benefits, medicinal properties and natural remedies of common foods and is a user-friendly reference guide for making healthy eating a lifelong habit.

The authors believe that consuming vegetables on a regular basis should be the primary focus of any healthy diet. Vegetables provide a wider range of nutrients than any other type of food including vitamins, minerals, carbohydrates and protein and are rich in phytonutrients which are associated with lowering the risk of cancer. To maximize nutritional intake, baking, steaming or lightly stir-frying vegetables is recommended. By boiling or overcooking vegetables, the vital nutrients and natural flavors are lost as they are leached into the water. Always choose fresh, organic produce if possible, with the next best option being frozen fruits and vegetables which contain far more nutrients than canned products. They emphasize consuming healthy nuts and seeds (almonds, Brazil nuts, flaxseeds, pecans, pumpkins, sunflower seeds, walnuts), whole grains (amaranth, barley, brown rice, millet, oats, quinoa, spelt, wheat), healthy oils (canola, coconut, flaxseed, macadamia, olive oil) and avoid oils with too much omega 6 fatty acids (corn, safflower, soy, sunflower). Although flaxseed oil is recommended, they advise not to cook with flaxseed oil because heat damages the omega 3 fatty acids. There are also certain types of foods they believe that should be completely avoided. These include white flour products (breads, cakes, muffins, pretzels), refined sugar products (baked goods, cereals, candies), processed foods with empty calories (canned foods, movie popcorn, potato chips), butter, margarine and shortening, smoked/cured meats (bacon, ham, hot dogs, luncheon meats, sausages, spam) and meat that is too charred or well done.

The authors have collaborated to illustrate their own version of a food pyramid with their appropriately named "Optimal Health Food Pyramid" illustrated on the following page. It combines the most advantageous health aspects of the Mediterranean and Asian Diet Pyramids, addresses the glycemic index of carbohydrates, promotes healthy oils and offers accurate serving sizes.

~ Optimal Health Food Pyramid ~

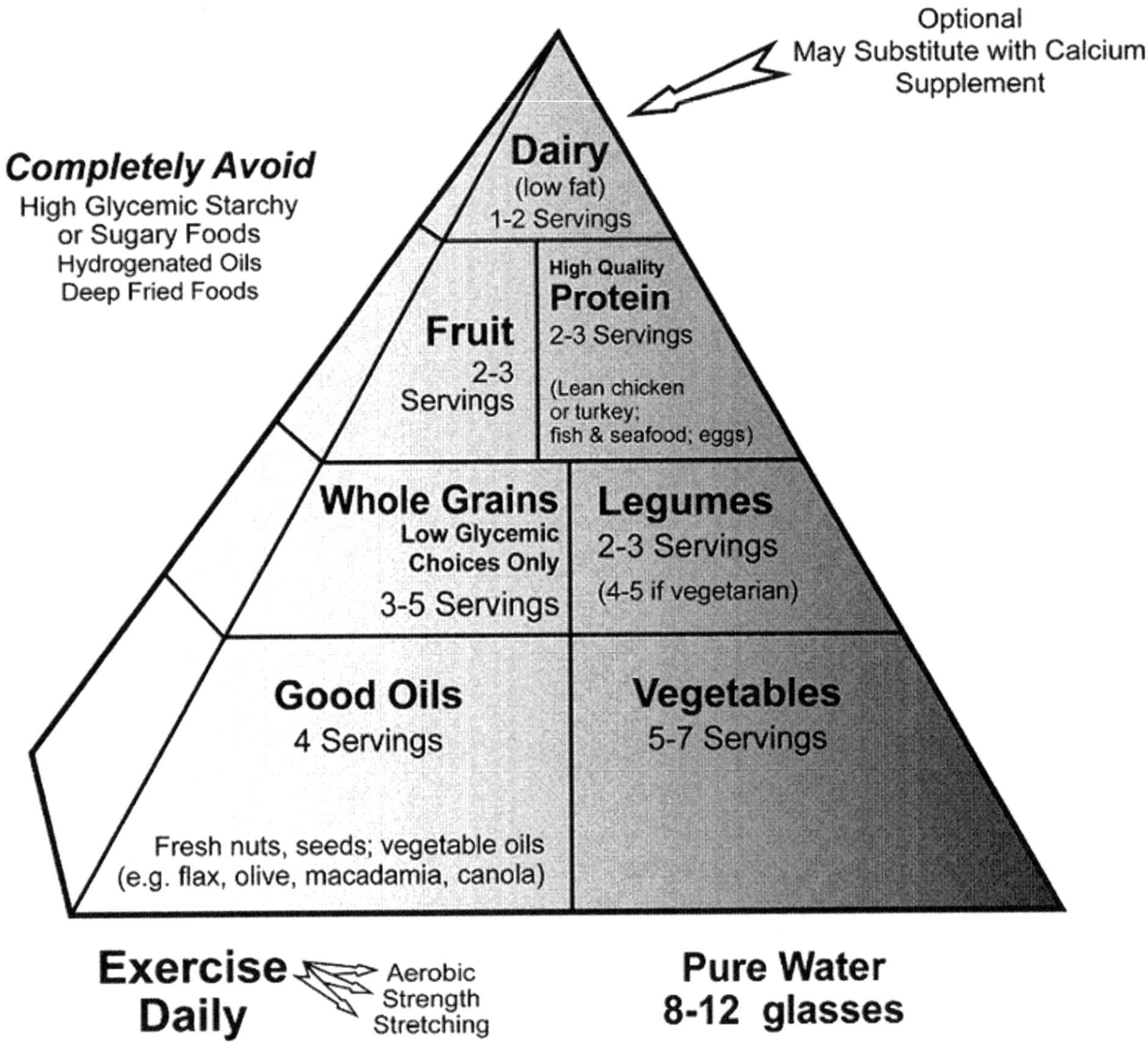

Remember!

Basic supplement program includes
High Potency Multivitamin/Mineral; Greens Drink; Fish Oils

~ Dietary Recommendations ~

In 1941, the U.S. Food and Nutrition Board of the National Academy of Sciences established standards for daily vitamin and mineral intake called Recommended Daily Allowances (RDA's) to assist in making smart food choices and adopting healthy eating practices. The Federal Nutrition Labeling and Education Act of 1992 sought to improve nutrition labeling on food products and created a new dietary reference term called Daily Value (DV). DV's are comprised of two nutritional references called the Daily Reference Values (DRV's) and the Reference Daily Intakes (RDI's). The DRV's relate to protein, fiber, fats, cholesterol, carbohydrates, potassium and sodium, and the RDI's are based on the former RDA standards for vitamins and mineral intake. Visible on modern day food labels, DV represents the percentage of nutrients obtained in one serving of food.

In 1998, the U.S. Food and Nutrition Board updated their dietary guidelines and changed the previous RDA standards to the *Dietary Reference Intake* (DRI) which is helpful for assessing and planning healthy diets by providing appropriate amounts of each nutrient. The DRI represents a group of nutritional references designed to optimize health including the updated RDA's as well as the Adequate Intake (AI) which applies when no RDA exists, Tolerable Upper Intake Level (UL) which is the maximum nutrient intake unlikely to increase risk of health adversities and Estimated Average Requirement (EAR) which is the average daily intake of a nutrient will meet the nutritional needs of half of the people in a group.

The U.S. Department of Agriculture (USDA) and the U.S. Department of Health and Human Services (DHHS) have created the "Dietary Guidelines for Americans" which are based on DRI values and are the foundation of federal nutrition policy and nutritional education. These guidelines promote healthy eating habits, advocate proper weight management through adequate exercise and inform the public about wholesome nutrition and its link to reducing the risk of many degenerative diseases. The following table lists vitamins and minerals with DV and DRI values for adult men and women adapted from the DRI reports. For more information on the Dietary Guidelines for Americans please visit www.cnpp.usda.gov/dietaryguidelines.htm, for the U.S. Food and Nutrition Board of the Institute of Medicine visit www.iom.edu, and for the National Academy of Sciences, visit www.nationalacademies.org.

Dietary Reference Intake DRI (RDA)

Vitamins	Daily Value (DV)	DRI (RDA) for adult Men	DRI (RDA) for adult Women
Vitamin A	5000 IU	3000 IU	2,3000 IU
Vitamin C	60 mg	90 mg	75 mg
Vitamin D	400 IU	600 IU	600 IU
Vitamin E	30 IU	30 IU	30 IU
Vitamin K	80 mcg	120 mcg (AI)	90 mcg (AI)
Choline	n/a	550 mg (AI)	425 mg (AI)
Thiamine (B1)	1.5 mg	1.2 mg	1.1 mg
Riboflavin (B2)	1.7 mg	1.3 mg	1.1 mg
Niacin (B3)	20 mg	16 mg	14 mg
Pantothenic Acid (B5)	10 mg	5 mg (AI)	5 mg (AI)
Pyridoxine (B6)	2 mg	1.3 mg	1.3 mg
Biotin (B7)	300 mcg	30 mcg (AI)	30 mcg (AI)
Folic Acid (B9)	400 mcg	400 mcg	400 mcg
Cyanocobalamin (B12)	6 mcg	2.4 mcg	2.4 mcg
Minerals	**Daily Value (DV)**	**DRI (RDA) for adult Men**	**DRI (RDA) for adult Women**
Calcium	1000 mg	1000 mg	1000-1200 mg
Chromium	120 mcg	35 mcg (AI)	25 mcg (AI)
Copper	2 mg	0.9 mg	0.9 mg
Iodine	150 mcg	150 mcg	150 mcg
Iron	18 mg	8 mg	18 mg
Magnesium	400 mg	420 mg	320 mg
Manganese	2 mg	2.3 mg (AI)	1.8 mg (AI)
Molybdenum	75 mcg	45 mcg	45 mcg
Phosphorus	1000 mg	700 mg	700 mg
Potassium	4000 mg	4700 mg (AI)	4700 mg (AI)
Selenium	70 mcg	55 mcg	55 mcg
Zinc	15 mg	11 mg	8 mg

*The RDA is given unless no RDA has been established, in which case Adequate Intake (AI) is indicated.

~ Wholesome Nutrition Table ~

Low-fat, nutrient-dense foods are the key to optimizing health and longevity. The following table illustrates the types of foods that are healthy to eat and those that are best to avoid.

Wholesome Nutrition Table		
Food Type	**Healthy Foods**	**Foods to Avoid**
Beans	all beans (except fava), organic, sprouted	canned beans with preservatives or salt, fava beans, pork and beans
Dairy	almond milk, cottage cheese, feta, kefir, mozzarella, rice milk, ricotta, skim milk, soy milk, yogurt (low-fat, non-fat, unsweetened)	artificially colored cheese, high-fat cheese (blue cheese, cheddar cheese, cream cheese), ice cream, pasteurized products
Eggs	organic, egg whites, free-range, hard boiled, poached, scrambled	fried, pickled, salted
Fish	halibut, mackerel, wild-caught salmon, freshwater whitefish, tuna fish (in water, limited)	anchovies, canned fish (in oil), fried fish, raw fish, salted fish, shellfish
Fruits	organic, fresh, unsweetened, locally grown, seasonal, stewed, frozen (unsweetened)	bottled, canned, processed, sweetened
Grains	whole grains (amaranth, barley, bran, brown rice, buckwheat, millet, oats, quinoa, wheat germ), whole grain bread/cereal/flour	instant cereal/oatmeal, white rice, white flour (biscuits, crackers, pancakes, pasta)
Meats	organic, free-range chicken/turkey, lean red meat (limited)	beef, gravies, hot dogs, luncheon meats, organ meats, pickled, pork, processed, smoked
Nuts/Seeds	raw, organic, unsalted	processed, roasted, salted, sugary
Oils	canola, corn, flaxseed, olive, safflower, sesame, soybean, sunflower	hardened oil, hydrogenated oil (trans fats), margarine, mayonnaise, processed oil, saturated fats, shortenings
Spices	cayenne pepper, cinnamon, dried herbs (all), garlic, ginger, miso, mustard, onions, sea salt, seaweed, tamari, turmeric	black pepper, white pepper, vinegar (except pure apple cider vinegar)
Sweets	barley malt, blackstrap molasses, honey (raw), maple syrup (pure), rice syrup, stevia	artificial sweeteners, brown sugar, candy, chocolate, corn syrup, jams, jellies, white sugar
Vegetables	raw, fresh, frozen (no salt/additives), locally grown, organic, seasonal	canned, processed, with additives or added salt

~ The Glycemic Index ~

When carbohydrates are digested, they break down and release sugar (glucose) into the blood stream. The glycemic index (GI) is a measure of how much carbohydrates will raise blood sugar levels as compared to white bread which has a maximum GI score of 100. A high GI score is 70 and above, a medium GI score is 56 - 69 and a low GI score is 55 and under. Foods on the lower end of the spectrum tend to have less of an effect on blood-sugar and only raise levels moderately; whereas foods in the medium to high range may cause blood sugar to rise more rapidly and possibly to unsafe levels. Since the glycemic index can help predict how our bodies will metabolize various carbohydrates into sugar, it is extremely helpful in managing diabetes as well as lowering blood pressure and cholesterol, promoting weight loss and increasing athletic endurance. The Glycemic Index is an international database developed by the Human Nutrition Unit, School of Molecular and Microbial Biosciences, University of Sydney. It provides research information, health news and nutritional calculations ranking carbohydrates and their impact on blood sugar levels. Below are foods categorized by their low, medium and high glycemic index scores. For more information, visit www.glycemicindex.com

Low GI score **(55 or less)** – almonds, apples, apricots (dried), artichokes, asparagus, barley, buckwheat, bulgur, beans (baked, black, garbanzo, kidney, lima, navy, pinto, red, soy), barley, bell peppers, bran, broccoli, cereals (all-bran and rice bran) cabbage, carrots (raw), cashews, cauliflower, celery, cherries, cucumber, grapefruit, grapes, jams, kiwi, legumes, lentils, lettuce, milk (fat-free, skim, semi-skimmed, whole), mushrooms, onions, oranges/orange juice, pasta (fettuccine, ravioli, vermicelli, spaghetti), peaches, peanuts, peanut butter, pears, peas, plums, prunes, quinoa, sourdough bread, soy foods (edamame, miso, tamari, tempeh, tofu, soy milk), spinach, sweet potatoes, strawberries, tomatoes, walnuts, whole grains, whole milk, yogurt, zucchini

Medium GI score **(56 – 69)** – apricots (canned), bananas, basmati rice, beets, brown rice, cantaloupe, carrots (cooked), cereals (cream of wheat, grape-nuts, mueslix, nutragrain, shredded wheat), couscous, cornmeal, croissant, figs, honey (raw), ice cream, macaroni and cheese, mangoes, oatmeal, papayas, pears, pineapples, pita bread, popcorn, potato chips, raisins, long-grain rice, rye bread, sweet corn, table sugar, wheat thins, wheat bread, wild rice

High GI score **(70 and above)** – bagels, baguette, carrots (caramelized), cereals (bran flakes, cheerios, corn flakes, grape-nut flakes, raisin bran, rice chex, rice krispies, total), corn chips, dates, doughnuts, fava beans, french bread, french fries, gatorade, graham crackers, jasmine rice, millet, parsnips, potatoes (baked, instant), pretzels, pumpkin, rice cakes/crackers, saltine crackers, spelt, tapioca, waffles, watermelon, white bread, white flour, white rice

~ The Living Colors of Fruits & Vegetables ~

Red fruits and vegetables – contain phytonutrients like hesperidin, lycopene and ellagic acid that reduce the risk of prostate cancer, lower blood pressure and cholesterol levels, inhibit tumor growth, neutralize free radicals and alleviate arthritis and inflammation.

Examples: beets, cherries, cranberries, guava, papayas, pink or red grapefruit, pomegranates, radishes, raspberries, red apples, red bell peppers, red chili peppers, red grapes, red onions, red pears, red potatoes, strawberries, tomatoes, watermelon

Orange and Yellow fruits and vegetables – contain beta-carotene, flavonoids, lycopene, potassium and vitamin C which reduces the risk of lung and prostate cancer, protects against macular degeneration, lowers blood pressure and cholesterol, promotes collagen formation, builds healthy bones and joints, eliminates free radicals and supports proper pH balance in the body.

Examples: apricots, cantaloupe, carrots, grapefruit, lemons, mangoes, nectarines, oranges, papayas, peaches, persimmons, pineapples, pumpkin, squash, sweet corn, sweet potatoes, tangerines, yellow apples, yellow pears, yellow bell peppers, yellow potatoes

Green vegetables and fruit – contain beta-carotene, calcium, chlorophyll, fiber, folate, lutein and vitamin C that reduces the risk of cancer, lowers blood pressure and cholesterol levels, normalizes digestion, improves vision and stimulates the immune system.

Examples: artichokes, arugula, asparagus, avocados, broccoli, Brussels sprouts, cabbage, celery, cucumber, endive, green apples, green beans, green grapes, green onion, green pears, green onions, honeydew, kiwi, leeks, lettuce, limes, okra, peas, spinach, watercress, zucchini

Blue and Purple fruits and vegetables – contain nutrients like lutein, vitamin C, fiber and flavonoids that improve vision, help lower blood pressure and cholesterol, strengthen the immune system, support healthy digestion, improve calcium and nutrient absorption and inhibits cancer cells.

Examples: black currants, blackberries, blueberries, dried plums, eggplant, grapes, plums, prunes, purple cabbage, purple figs, purple grapes, purple potatoes, raisins

White fruits and vegetables – contain antioxidants, phytonutrients, potassium, antibacterial nutrients like *allicin* that strengthen the immune system, maintain healthy cholesterol and hormone levels and reduces the risk of breast, colon, prostate and hormone-related cancers.

Examples: artichokes, bananas, brown pears, cauliflower, dates, garlic, ginger, jicama, mushrooms, onions, parsnips, potatoes, shallots, turnips, white corn, white nectarines, white peaches

~ The pH of Food ~

When we are born our bodies have an ideal pH balance, yet as we age our bodies become increasingly acidic. Many nutritional experts believe the key to preventative health is to eat raw, natural foods that keep the body within a normal pH range. The diet should consist of 75-80% alkaline-forming foods and about 20-25% acid-forming foods. The acidity or alkalinity of food is measured by the pH value of the ash residue that remains after food has been ingested and metabolized. This residue can be alkaline, acidic or neutral depending on the mineral content of the food. Calcium, magnesium, potassium, iron, sodium and zinc leave an alkaline residue while phosphorous, sulfur, chlorine and iodine tend to leave an acidic residue. Alkaline-forming foods include: most vegetables and fruits (raw), aloe vera juice, green tea, herbs/spices (most), honey (raw), millet, mushrooms, nuts (almonds, Brazil nuts, chestnuts), onions, raisins, seeds (flax, pumpkin, sesame, sunflower), soy beans, sprouts and whey. Acid-forming foods include: alcohol, artificial sweeteners, beans (most), black tea, coffee, dairy, some fruits (blueberries, cranberries, plums, prunes, sour cherries), grains (most), herbs/spices (black pepper, mustard, soy sauce), legumes, lentils, meats, molasses, nuts/seeds (most), olives, sugar & white flour.

The rather confusing part about pH and food is in regards to fruit. The acid or alkaline-forming tendency of food in the body has little to do with the pH of food itself. Lemons and limes are great examples because they are very acidic as you eat them; however the ash residue they leave behind after digestion is alkaline so lemons and limes are considered alkaline-forming foods. Many health disorders such as arthritis, cancer, diabetes, obesity and osteoporosis are associated with an acidic body environment. Besides eating raw, alkaline-forming foods, exercising and breathing oxygen deep into the lungs have alkalizing effects on the body as well.

Acidic					Neutral				Alkaline	
> 4.5	5	5.5	6	6.5	7	7.5	8	8.5	9	9.5 <

The pH scale goes from 0 to 14, with 7 being neutral and is the natural pH of water. Below 7 is considered acidic and above 7 is considered alkaline. The blood, lymph and spinal fluid of the human body is slightly alkaline with a pH of 7.4 which is the ideal pH level for a healthy human body. The heart circulates blood and physical exercise circulates lymph; a clear liquid that tissues depend on to provide oxygen and nutrients to the cells and carry off waste material. If the lymph substance does not circulate in the body, cells and tissues become more acidic, saturate with toxins and create a disease-friendly environment. There are now saliva and urine tests available to monitor pH levels.

~ Detoxification ~

The body accumulates many toxins from various air, food and water sources throughout our lifetime which may lead to poor health. Whether it's agricultural chemicals (herbicides, insecticides, pesticides), processed foods, household cleaners, lead from old house paint, medications, second-hand smoke, smog or tap water…toxins are all around us. Our digestive system has to filter out harmful toxins on a daily basis through the bowel, kidneys, liver, lungs and skin. Feeling tired, low-energy, having slow or cloudy thinking, being constipated and/or feeling bloated are all good indications of toxins accumulating in the body. During a detoxification program, harmful toxins are released back into the bloodstream in order to be expelled. For many people it may cause temporary flu-like symptoms or an upset stomach. If toxins are not fully flushed out, they can easily reattach to other parts of the body and continue their damage. This is why it is imperative to drink plenty of water during detoxification.

The main focus of detoxification is easing into the program, as well as keeping toxin levels as low as possible which can be achieved by several methods. A great way to start is by maintaining a high-fiber diet, reducing stress, exercising, sweating and drinking plenty of distilled water with lemon. Eat plenty of raw foods, fresh organic vegetables, onions, garlic and ginger, and cleanse the liver by drinking aloe vera juice and decaffeinated green tea. Other beneficial foods include amaranth, barley, beans, brown rice, buckwheat, cayenne pepper, ginger, kelp, nuts/seeds (raw), oats (raw), oils (flaxseed, hempseed, olive, sesame and walnut), quinoa, rice milk, salmon (wild-caught), tahini, tofu, whole grains and wild rice. Vitamins A, C & E, selenium and zinc are essential for eliminating toxins from the body. There are also natural detox supplements like benonite, CoQ10, flaxseed oil, gingko biloba, grape seed extract, milk thistle and red clover that have shown to be quite effective. Massage therapy is a great option because it releases toxins that are stored in muscle tissue, increases blood flow and improves cardiovascular health. A natural colon-cleanse product like psyllium is very effective at flushing out toxins and waste that build up along the walls of the digestive tract.

A hot Epsom salt bath is another effective, natural way to flush toxins out of the body. Combined with hot water, it draws toxins out of the body to the skin's surface for removal. Epsom salt baths help to alleviate pain by reducing stiffness and swelling, and also helps remove lactic-acid that builds up in muscles from working out and/or playing sports. Because it is so effective, many professional athletes soak in Epsom salt baths after games and workouts so they can be physically ready to perform the next day while being as pain-free as possible. *Foods to avoid while detoxing: alcohol, chocolate, coffee, dairy, fermented foods, meats, peanuts, shellfish, sugar, vinegar and yeast.*

~ Mercury Content of Fish & Shellfish ~

Fish and shellfish are rich sources of high-quality protein, minerals, omega 3's and are low in saturated fat, yet nearly all contain some traces of mercury. The risk of obtaining excessive amounts of mercury depends on the levels of mercury in the fish and the amount of fish consumed. "Wild-caught" salmon has little to no mercury content, whereas salmon raised in fisheries often contain much higher levels of mercury. Shellfish are bottom feeders and often contain low to moderate levels of mercury as well.

The Environmental Protection Agency (EPA) publishes recommendations about fish consumption and correlating health benefits. Shark, swordfish, king mackerel etc. are not recommended due to high mercury content. Albacore tuna is known to contain high levels of mercury as well so limited consumption is suggested. Low-mercury fish include wild-caught salmon, shrimp, pollock and catfish, low-moderate mercury levels in canned light tuna. Pregnant women should avoid and/or use extreme caution when consuming any fish or fish oil supplements due to possible mercury content. The United States Food and Drug Administration (FDA) has a monitoring program that records mercury concentrations in fish, and publishes risk and benefit assessment reports in regards to commercial fish consumption. Below is a listing of common fish and shellfish according to their mercury content. For more information, please visit www.fda.gov and www.epa.gov.

Mercury Content of Fish & Shellfish			
Low Mercury Content		**Moderate Mercury Content**	**High Mercury Content**
Anchovies	Perch	Bass	Bluefish
Carp	Pollock	Cod	Grouper
Catfish	Salmon	Halibut	Marlin
Clam	Sardines	Lobster	Orange Roughy
Crab	Scallop	Mackerel	Sea Bass
Crawfish	Shrimp	Mahi Mahi	Shark
Flounder	Sole	Monkfish	Swordfish
Haddock	Tilapia	Perch	Tilefish
Herring	Trout	Snapper	Tuna (Ahi, Yellowfin)
Oyster	Whitefish	Tuna (canned chunk light)	Tuna (canned Albacore)

~ Pesticide Content of Fruits & Vegetables ~

Founded in 1993 by Ken Cook and Richard Wiles, the Environmental Working Group (EWG) is a non-profit organization and a consumer advocate group comprised of experts spanning various industries including engineers, scientists, lawyers and policy experts to find solutions to modern day health and environmental issues. EWG provides helpful resources to protect consumers from health disorders attributed to various toxic contaminants while pushing for policy change. The "EWG's 2010 Shoppers Guide to Pesticides" scores vegetables and fruits based upon their pesticide contaminant levels. Specific crops were chosen as a result of a USDA food consumption analysis and were ranked on a combined score of six different categories of contamination measurements with peaches containing the highest levels and sweet corn with the lowest. For more information, please visit www.ewg.org

Pesticide Content of Vegetables & Fruits			
Foods	**Combined Score**	**Foods**	**Combined Score**
Peaches	100	Kale	39
Strawberries	89	Mushrooms	36
Apples	88	Cantaloupe	36
Spinach	85	Sweet Potatoes	35
Nectarines	85	Grapefruit	34
Celery	83	Winter Squash	34
Pears	80	Blueberries	30
Cherries	76	Watermelon	27
Potatoes	67	Plums	26
Bell Peppers	66	Tangerines	25
Raspberries	66	Cabbage	25
Carrots	57	Papayas	23
Green Beans	57	Kiwi	23
Hot Peppers	55	Bananas	19
Oranges	53	Broccoli	18
Apricots	51	Onions	17
Cucumbers	51	Asparagus	16
Tomatoes	48	Sweet Peas	13
Collard Greens	48	Mango	12
Grapes	47	Cauliflower	10
Turnip Greens	41	Pineapples	6
Honeydew Melons	40	Avocados	4
Lettuce	40	Sweet Corn	1

~ Intestinal Parasites ~

This might come as a shock, but approximately 80% of people have some sort of parasitic infection in their digestive system. From cysts in the blood, to pinworms, whipworms, hookworms and tapeworms several feet long, an intestinal parasite is an organism that lives inside the human gastrointestinal tract which acts as a host for the invader. Parasites are dependent upon their hosts because they are unable to produce food for themselves and survive on their own. They are harmful to humans because they strip our bodies of vital nutrients, eat away at our tissues and cells and create a toxic environment in our body that makes people ill. Intestinal parasites usually enter the body through the skin or mouth and can permeate through intestinal walls to invade other organs.

Since intestinal parasites can live inside the human body for years without their presence being known, they are far more common than you might think. The main factors for contracting intestinal parasites include biting fingernails, contact with children, improper food handling, inhaling airborne eggs, insect bites, lack of personal hygiene, contact with pets, poor diet, eating pork, poor sanitation (especially at day care centers and mental health institutions), poorly cleaned lettuce and/or vegetables, undercooked or raw meat (sushi), tap water, well water, traveling abroad and walking barefoot in dirt. There are so many ways to get these parasites it is simply disturbing!

The most common symptoms include abdominal pain, anal itching, bloating, bronchitis, chest pain, constipation, congestion, cough, diarrhea, fever, frequent colds/flu, heart burn, insomnia, loss of weight with continual hunger, low energy, muscle damage, skin rashes, restlessness, stomach pain and digestive rumbling that is unrelated to hunger. There are many types of parasite cleanses available at local health food stores. Some of the herbs contained in these cleanses may be harsh on the digestive tract so use caution, know your allergies and never combine with any medications. Below is a list of foods, herbs and supplements that help fight off these intestinal invaders. *What have you got to lose?*

Anti-Parasitic Nutrition – **Foods:** beets, brown rice, cabbage, carrots, cranberries, figs, grapefruit juice, horseradish, leafy green vegetables, lemons, limes, onions, papayas, peaches, pineapples, pomegranate juice, pumpkin seeds, radishes, sesame seeds, sweet potato, squash, wasabi, whole grains; **Spices:** cayenne pepper, fennel, garlic, ginger, oregano, parsley, rosemary, sage, thyme, turmeric; **Supplements:** (vitamins B-complex & C, iron, zinc), acidophilus, aloe vera juice, bentonite, bromelain, coconut oil, echinacea, flaxseed oil, grapefruit seed extract, graviola, psyllium, **Herbs:** black cohosh, black walnut, cascara sagrada, chamomile, chaparral, clove, epazote, goldenseal, licorice, mullein, pau d' arco, slippery elm, valerian, wood betony, wormwood

***Parasite cleanses should be avoided by pregnant and nursing women!**

~ Health and Nutrition Tips ~

Aging – remain active, maintain lean body mass, moderate stretching, low-impact exercise, read as much as possible, listen to uplifting music, paint/draw, keep a journal, spend time with loved ones, consider a small pet, get plenty of sleep, take naps when tired, practice deep breathing, eat organic foods, drink plenty of water, quit smoking and drinking alcohol and never take excessive medications

Butter vs. Margarine – margarine contains higher amounts of unsaturated 'good' fats, but also contains hydrogenated oils or 'trans-fats' which may lead to high blood pressure and cardiovascular disease, is chemically processed to increase shelf life and has minimal nutritional content. Butter contains more saturated 'bad' fats which may increase cholesterol; however using butter that is low in saturated fat may be a much healthier option for some

Caffeine (the good and the bad) – **good:** stimulates metabolism and the central nervous system, increases alertness, enhances athletic performance, reduces the risk of gallstones, cirrhosis and Parkinson's, helps prevent dental cavities; **bad:** increases blood pressure, insomnia, anxiety, arthritis and inhibits the absorption of calcium and iron

Chelated Supplements – the *chelation* process binds molecules together which increases the absorption of nutrients

Common Signs of Cancer – frequent coughing, difficulty swallowing, change in bowel/bladder function, indigestion, sores that won't heal, unusual bleeding, lump or thickening of skin, change in mole or wart; common anti-cancer foods and spices are: basil, beans, beets, berries, broccoli, cabbage, garlic, ginger, onions, oregano, parsley, spinach, sweet potatoes, tomatoes, turmeric, whole grains

Deep Breathing – proper breathing is necessary for longevity, deep breathing in through the nose increases necessary amounts of oxygen the brain needs to function properly, detoxifies the lungs, stimulates metabolism, increases energy, improves body posture and increases quality of sleep

Digestive Food Combos – vegetables and meats, and vegetables and carbohydrates are good digestive food combinations; carbohydrates are easier to digest when eaten alone or with vegetables, meats and carbohydrates clash digestively because proteins need acids and carbohydrates need alkalinity to digest properly (fish & chips, meat & potatoes are common food combos but may inhibit digestion)

Digestive Health – chewing slowly helps break down food into smaller particles for easier digestion and better absorption of nutrients, eat smaller meal portions especially at night, stop eating as soon as stomach feels full, eat at least 3-4 hours before going to sleep to allow for proper digestion

Fruits – fruits should be eaten between or separate from meals, do not digest well with grains; consume early in the day to burn off natural sugars and carbohydrates (eat veggies the rest of the day)

Gluten-Free Foods – gluten is a protein found in certain grains like barley, bulgur, couscous, durum, kamut, miso, oats, rye, spelt, wheat & wheat products, and should be avoided by those who are gluten intolerant (Celiac disease); recommended foods for a gluten-free diet include: alfalfa, almonds, amaranth, apple cider vinegar, artichokes, balsamic vinegar, basmati rice, brown rice, buckwheat, chicken, corn, cottage cheese, custard, eggs, fish, flaxseed, fruits, garbanzo beans, herbal tea, honey (raw), kudzu, legumes, lentils, long-grain rice, millet, molasses, quinoa, rice bran, rice cakes, sago, sesame, soy foods, sunflower seeds, sweet potatoes, tapioca, taro flour, vegetables, water chestnuts

Lactose-Free Milk – almond, rice and soy milk are available for those who are lactose-intolerant and/or who prefer not to drink cow's milk due possible hormone and steroid injections, all are rich in calcium, magnesium and other essential minerals, usually organic, hormone and steroid free; soy milk provides protein and is low in saturated fat, but consuming too much may lower good (HDL) cholesterol levels

Natural Sweeteners – artificial sweeteners like aspartame and saccharin may be unhealthful by creating toxins in the body and possibly interfering with blood sugar levels; natural sweeteners to consider are: agave nectars, barley malt, brown rice syrup, honey (raw), maple syrup, molasses, stevia and xylitol

Organic Foods – Organic foods are grown naturally without pesticides, herbicides, insecticides or any other chemicals, organic soil has a higher concentration of micronutrients and has double the nutrients of non-organic foods, fresher tasting than non-organic foods, may have shorter shelf life

Overcooking – over-cooking foods destroys enzymes and nutrients; steaming is recommended because it keeps nutrients inside, also lightly cook, poach or stir-fry vegetables, always cook meat until there is no redness, avoid carcinogens from eating charred or burnt meat from the grill, use sea salt only, soak/sprout beans for increased nutrition and easier digestion

Overeating – most of the toxins we accumulate come from food; overeating produces high levels of toxins, excess fat, arthritis and muscle pain, is linked to hormonal imbalances, speeds up aging, raises blood sugar and triglyceride levels, increases the risk of cancer, diabetes, cardiovascular disease, impotence, infertility, depression, increases weight, slows down metabolism and lowers energy levels

Sea Salt – unlike refined table salt, sea salt is made from evaporated seawater, is naturally unrefined to increase its bio-availability and is nutritionally abundant, is a healthier salt substitute and is easy to absorb, has traces of essentially every mineral known, excess amounts of table salt may lead to high blood pressure, mineral deficiencies and other health disorders

Seasonal Foods – eating a variety of the freshest foods at the peak of each harvest helps maximize nutritional intake; *Spring* provides leafy green vegetables, basil and parsley; *Summer* harvests include berries, kiwi, melons, nectarines, peaches and watermelon, vegetables include broccoli, cauliflower and squash, meats include chicken and fish; *Autumn* calls for more ginger, onions, turkey and sweet potatoes; *Winter* foods include beef, eggs and vegetables like carrots, corn, garlic, onions and potatoes

Sleep – sleep is the key to energy, vitality and longevity, improves the digestive and nervous system, detoxifies the body, repairs damaged tissues, reduces stress and depression, increases cardiovascular health; calcium & chamomile tea are great for inducing sleep - alcohol, caffeine & sugar disrupt sleep

Tongue Scraping – great for cleaning toxins out of the mouth that accumulate during sleep and create plaque; use in the morning before brushing your teeth - most dentists will supply these

Vegetarian Diet – consider a high-fiber diet that consist of fruits, vegetables, whole grains, legumes, nuts and seeds; may be difficult to maintain adequate protein intake, some need to supplement B6, B12, iron and zinc or obtain them from fortified foods

Part Four

Common Health Disorders

~ Common Health Disorders ~

This section addresses and defines the most common types of health disorders that people suffer from today. Highlighted are the possible factors, common symptoms and relative nutrition that may be helpful in improving health conditions. Know your allergies, and always check with your doctor before taking any new herbs, supplements or nutritional products that are unfamiliar to you.

Acidosis – *(body's pH level becomes overly acidic which may increase the risk of various digestive, respiratory and physical disorders)*

Possible Factors – acidic foods (beans, chocolate, dairy, fish, cereals/grains, meat, nuts) adrenal disorders, alcohol, aspirin, caffeine, coffee, excessive protein, excessive vitamin C, fried/fatty/spicy foods, inactivity, obesity, smoking, stomach ulcers, stress, sugar, white flour

Common Symptoms – arthritis, bad breath, bloating, constipation, diarrhea, excessive perspiration, flatulence, heartburn, indigestion, insomnia, loss of appetite, low blood pressure, migraines, nausea, osteoporosis, shortness of breath, vomiting

Helpful Nutrition – **Foods:** alfalfa sprouts, almonds, apples, apricots, avocados, bananas, beets, blackberries, broccoli, cabbage, cantaloupe, carrots, cauliflower, celery, chestnuts, cucumber, dates, eggplant, figs, grapes, grapefruit, kale, leafy green vegetables, leeks, lemons, limes, mangoes, melons, millet, mineral water w/ lemon, mushrooms, nectarines, onions, oranges, papayas, peaches, pears, pineapples, potato skins, pumpkin seeds, raisins, sesame seeds, spinach, strawberries, sweet potatoes, watercress, watermelon; **Spices:** cilantro, cinnamon, fennel, garlic, ginger, mustard, parsley, turmeric; **Supplements:** (vitamins A & B, calcium, magnesium, phosphorus, potassium), aloe vera juice, apple cider vinegar, flaxseed oil, grapefruit seed extract, wheatgrass juice; **Herbs:** dandelion, elder, hops

---

Acne – *(skin pores become clogged and inflamed from overactive oil glands)*

Possible Factors – alcohol, allergies, butter, caffeine, cheese, chocolate, dirty skin, fried/fatty/salty foods, hormone imbalance, makeup, nuts (most), processed foods, soft drinks, stress, sugar, white flour

Common Symptoms – blackheads, blemishes, cysts, lesions, nodules, oily/shiny skin, pustules, red bumps, scarring, whiteheads

Helpful Nutrition – **Foods:** alfalfa sprouts, almonds, beets, brown rice, cashews, grapes (red), leafy green vegetables, lentils, oat bran, pineapples, soybeans, soy milk, strawberries, sunflower seeds, Swiss chard, vegetables (raw), whole grains; **Spices:** cayenne pepper, garlic; **Supplements:** (vitamins A, B-complex, C, D & E, chromium, potassium, selenium, zinc), acidophilus, aloe vera juice, apple cider vinegar (topically), chlorophyll, echinacea, flaxseed oil, milk thistle, royal jelly, saw palmetto, wheatgrass juice; **Herbs:** burdock, dandelion, lavender, Oregon grape, red clover

Adrenal Gland Disorders (Addison's disease) – *(autoimmune disorder characterized by the immune system attacking the adrenal glands)*

Possible Factors – anemia, diabetes, heredity, hypothyroidism, inflammation, medications, poor diet, stress, sugar, weakened immune system, white flour

Common Symptoms – allergies, blood-sugar imbalance, cold feeling, depression, discoloration of skin, dizziness, fatigue, headaches, loss of appetite, low blood pressure, memory loss, more body hair, muscle weakness, nausea, red marks, salty-food cravings, weakened immune system

Helpful Nutrition – **Foods:** almonds, apples, bananas, barley, beans (kidney, lima), bell peppers (green & red), berries, broccoli, brown rice, Brussels sprouts, cabbage, carrots, cauliflower, cantaloupe, cherries, fruit juices (organic), grapefruit, hazelnuts, kale, leafy green vegetables, legumes, millet, molasses, mushrooms (shiitake), nuts, olive oil, onions, oranges, peaches, pineapples, salmon, sunflower seeds, tomatoes, tuna, whole grains; **Spices:** garlic, parsley, thyme; **Supplements:** (vitamins A, B-complex, C & E, calcium, chromium, magnesium, potassium, selenium, zinc), brewer's yeast, chlorophyll, coconut oil, CoQ10, cordyceps, fish oil, flaxseed oil, ginseng, lecithin, milk thistle, royal jelly, St. John's wort, wheatgrass juice; **Herbs:** ashwagandha, astragalus, borage, chuchuhuasi, primrose

---

Aging (premature) – *(decline of new cell production to replace old, damaged cells)*

Possible Factors – alcohol, amphetamines, caffeine, environmental/industrial toxins, heredity, overexposure to the sun, poor diet, smoking, stress, sugar, white flour

Common Symptoms – brittle bones, depression, disorientation, fatigue, hearing/memory/vision impairment, whitening hair, wrinkles

Helpful Nutrition – **Foods:** almonds, apples, barley, beans, bell peppers, berries, broccoli, cabbage, cantaloupe, carrots, cauliflower, celery, chia seeds, grapes (red), green tea (decaf), herring, kale, kefir, leafy green vegetables, lemons, limes, mangoes, mangosteen, mushrooms (shiitake), nectarines, nuts/seeds (raw), oats, onions, oranges, papayas, peaches, pomegranates, quinoa, salmon, soy foods, spinach, sweet potatoes, tuna, whole grains, zucchini; **Spices:** cayenne pepper, dill, fennel, garlic, ginger, parsley, thyme, turmeric; **Supplements:** (vitamins A, B-complex, C, D & E, boron, calcium, chromium, iron, magnesium, potassium, selenium, zinc), acidophilus, aloe vera juice, bentonite, coconut oil, CoQ10, cordyceps, fish oil, flaxseed oil, ginkgo biloba, ginseng, grape seed extract, milk thistle, psyllium, royal jelly, wheatgrass juice; **Herbs:** bilberry, burdock, licorice, nettle, red clover, yerba mate

---

AIDS/HIV (Acquired Immune Deficiency Syndrome / Human Immunodeficiency Virus) – *(the inability of the immune system to defend itself against infection and/or disease)*

Possible Factors – blood transfusions, heredity, intravenous drug use, unprotected sex

Common Symptoms – chronic coughing, constipation, dehydration, diarrhea, excessive perspiration, fatigue, fever, fibromyalgia, headache, loss of appetite, nausea, skin lesions, sore throat, swollen glands, trouble breathing, vomiting, weight loss

Helpful Nutrition – **Foods:** apples, artichokes, avocados, bananas, barley, beans, beets, beet greens, bell peppers, berries, broccoli, brown rice, Brussels sprouts, cabbage, carrots, cauliflower, chicken (skinless), green tea (decaf), kelp, lemons, limes, melons, millet, mushrooms (maitake, reishi, shiitake), nuts/seeds (raw), oat bran, olive oil, onions, oranges, papayas, peaches, pineapples, pumpkin, salmon, squash, sweet potatoes, tomatoes (cooked), whole grains, yogurt (low/non-fat); **Spices:** cayenne pepper, garlic; **Supplements:** (vitamins A, B-complex, C, D & E, germanium, selenium, zinc), aloe vera juice, coconut oil, CoQ10, cordyceps, echinacea, fish oil, ginkgo biloba, ginseng, grape seed extract, grapefruit seed extract, milk thistle, psyllium, royal jelly, St. John's wort, wheatgrass juice; **Herbs:** chaparral, licorice, pau d'arco, red clover

---

Alcoholism – *(progressive disorder marked by a chronic physiological and/or psychological dependence on alcohol)*

Possible Factors – anxiety, depression, family issues, heredity, social acceptance, stress

Common Symptoms – aggression, amnesia, anger, cardiovascular decline, cirrhosis, disorientation, drinking alone, high blood pressure, irregular heartbeat, lack of coordination, loss of interest, memory loss, mood swings, osteoporosis, relationship/family problems, seizures, stroke, sweating, violence

Helpful Nutrition – **Foods:** alfalfa sprouts, beans, berries, bran, broccoli, brown rice, cabbage, cantaloupe, carrot juice, cauliflower, collard greens, green tea (decaf), kelp, leafy green vegetables, lemons, lentils, oatmeal, onions, quinoa, salmon, soy foods, whole grains; **Spices:** cayenne pepper, garlic, turmeric; **Supplements:** (vitamins A, B-complex, C & E, calcium, magnesium, selenium, zinc), acidophilus, aloe vera juice, CoQ10, flaxseed oil, grape seed extract; **Herbs:** kudzu, passionflower, primrose, red clover, skullcap

---

Alkalosis – *(body's pH level becomes overly alkaline, far less common than acidosis)*

Possible Factors – antacids, diarrhea, excessive sodium, high cholesterol, nutritional deficiencies, ulcer medication

Common Symptoms – allergies, asthma, bone spur, bruising, coughing, cramps, high blood pressure, hyperventilation, hypothermia, indigestion, itching, menstrual disorders, muscle spasms, nausea, numbness, seizures, sleepiness, sore muscles and joints, vomiting

Helpful Nutrition – **Foods:** asparagus (tips), barley, beans, blueberries, breads, brown rice, Brussels sprouts, buckwheat, buttermilk, cashews, cheese, cherries (sour), chicken, cooked foods, cornstarch, cranberries, eggs, fish, kamut, legumes, lentils, milk, oats (raw), olives, organ meats, pasta, peanuts, pistachios, plums, prunes, rhubarb, salmon, sauerkraut, turkey, tuna, walnuts, whole grains, yogurt; **Supplements:** (vitamins B-complex, C, D, E & K, CoQ10, selenium)

Allergies – *(abnormal reaction of the immune system to certain foreign substances or foods)*

Possible Factors – alcohol, animal dander/hair, artificial coloring (Yellow No. 5 dye), bananas, beef, caffeine, chocolate, citrus fruit, cleaning chemicals, corn, cosmetics, dairy, dust, eggs, environmental toxins, fish, heredity, insect venom, MSG, mold, nitrates, oats, peanuts, pollen, pork, ragweed, shellfish, smoking, soy foods, strawberries, sugar, sulfites, tomatoes, tree nuts (almonds, Brazil nuts, cashews, chestnuts, hazelnuts, pecans, pistachios, walnuts), wheat, white rice, yeast

Common Symptoms – acid imbalance, coughing, diarrhea, dizzy spells, ear noises, eye discomfort, fatigue, fluid retention, headache, hives, hyperactivity, itching, memory loss, nasal congestion, rashes, sensitivity to light, shortness of breath, wheezing

Helpful Nutrition – **Foods:** apples, berries, broccoli, brown rice, cabbage, chicken, onions, sesame seeds, sweet potatoes, turkey; **Spices:** cayenne pepper, peppermint, thyme; **Supplements:** (vitamins A, B-complex, C & E, calcium, magnesium, manganese, potassium, selenium, zinc), acidophilus, aloe vera juice, apple cider vinegar, bromelain, CoQ10, flaxseed oil, grape seed extract, wheatgrass juice; **Herbs:** boswellia, dandelion, fenugreek, goldenseal, licorice, mullein, nettle, pau d'arco, yerba mate

---

Alzheimer's Disease – *(degenerative brain disorder associated with severe memory loss and/or disorientation)*

Possible Factors – alcohol, aluminum & mercury toxicity, arteriosclerosis/atherosclerosis, cured meats, environmental toxins, head trauma, heredity, high blood pressure, hypothyroidism, immune system malfunction, vitamin D deficiency, smoking, sodium nitrites

Common Symptoms – disorientation, impaired judgment, language difficulty, memory loss, misplacing items, mood swings, personality changes

Helpful Nutrition – **Foods:** apples, asparagus, avocados, beans, beets, bell peppers, blackberries, blueberries, broccoli, brown rice, Brussels sprouts, cabbage (red), cantaloupe, carrots, collard greens, green tea (decaf), grapefruit, grapes (red), herring, kale, kelp, kiwi, leafy green vegetables, lemons, limes, mackerel, mangoes, oat bran, onions, orange juice, pineapples, plums, pomegranates, pumpkin seeds, raspberries, rice bran, salmon (baked), sardines, sesame seeds, spinach, sweet potatoes, strawberries, sunflower seeds, whole grains; **Spices:** cayenne pepper, cinnamon, cumin, garlic, ginger, mustard, oregano, rosemary, sage, turmeric; **Supplements:** (vitamins A, B-complex, C, D & E, boron, calcium, choline, iron, magnesium, potassium, selenium, silicon, zinc), aloe vera juice, apple cider vinegar, chia seeds, coconut oil, CoQ10, fish oil, ginkgo biloba, ginseng, grape seed extract, lecithin, royal jelly, wheatgrass juice; **Herbs:** blessed thistle, butcher's broom, eyebright, primrose, valerian

<u>Anemia</u> – *(lack of red blood cells necessary for transporting oxygen from the lungs to the body)*

<u>Possible Factors</u> – bone marrow disease, cirrhosis, copper and iron deficiency, drug abuse, hemorrhoids, heredity, hormone imbalance, inflammation, menstrual bleeding, metal toxicity, oxalic acid-foods (almonds, cashews, chocolate, kale, nuts, soda, spinach, Swiss chard), smoking, sugar, ulcers, white flour

<u>Common Symptoms</u> – arthritis, coldness, constipation, depression, fatigue, headaches, irritability, loss of appetite, loss of libido, mouth sores, poor concentration, weakness

<u>Helpful Nutrition</u> – **Foods:** alfalfa sprouts, apples, apricots, asparagus, bananas, beans (kidney, lima, pinto), beetroot juice, beets, bell peppers, broccoli, cantaloupe, carrots, dates, egg yolks, figs, kale, kelp, leafy green vegetables, lentils, liver, mangoes, miso, molasses, mustard greens, okra, papayas, peaches, plums, prunes, raisins, salmon, squash, sweet potatoes, tempeh, walnuts, whole grains (except bran); **Spices:** cumin, fennel, parsley; **Supplements:** (vitamins B-complex & C, cobalt, copper, iron, molybdenum), brewer's yeast, chlorophyll, ginseng, royal jelly, spirulina, wheatgrass juice; **Herbs:** bilberry, dandelion, goldenseal, hawthorn, mullein, nettle, Oregon grape, pau d'arco, yellow dock

---

<u>Anorexia</u> – *(psychological eating disorder marked by self-starvation and severe weight loss)*

<u>Possible Factors</u> – alcohol, chemical imbalance, depression, drug abuse, fear of gaining weight, negative self-image, refusal to eat

<u>Common Symptoms</u> – coldness, continuous dieting, dehydration, denial, dizziness, excessive exercising, food obsession, irregular heartbeat, low blood pressure, physical weakness, protruding bones, rapid drop in weight, ulcers

<u>Helpful Nutrition</u> – **Foods:** apples, apricots, artichokes, baked potatoes, bananas, beans, blueberries, bran, cantaloupe, carrots, corn, dates, figs, fruit juices (organic), leafy green vegetables, lentils, mangoes, nuts/seeds (raw), oatmeal, pears, peas, pomegranate juice, raisins, salmon, soy foods, strawberries, sweet potatoes, whole grains; **Spices:** cumin, fennel, ginger, mustard, peppermint; **Supplements:** (vitamins B-complex, C, D & E, calcium, magnesium, potassium, selenium, zinc), acidophilus, brewer's yeast, flaxseed oil, ginseng, milk thistle; **Herbs:** blessed thistle

---

<u>Anxiety</u> – *(malfunction in brain chemistry causing unexpected episodes of fear, stress and/or apprehensiveness)*

<u>Possible Factors</u> – alcohol, caffeine, food allergies, heights, hypoglycemia, loneliness, multiple sclerosis (MS), natural disaster or death, poor diet, public places, smoking, sugar

Common Symptoms – claustrophobic sensations, confusion, decreased libido, dizziness, excessive perspiration, headaches, hot flashes, increased heart rate, insomnia, lack of concentration, mood swings, muscle stiffness or twitching, nightmares, panic attacks, shortness of breath, trembling, stress

Helpful Nutrition – **Foods:** apricots, asparagus, avocados, bananas, beans, broccoli, brown rice, chicken, leafy green vegetables, lentils, molasses, nuts/seeds (raw), oats (raw), salmon, tofu, whole grains, yogurt; **Spices:** fennel, garlic, peppermint; **Supplements:** (vitamins B-complex, C, E, calcium, chromium, magnesium, molybdenum, selenium, zinc), apple cider vinegar, brewer's yeast, coconut oil, fish oil, ginseng, milk thistle, royal jelly; **Herbs:** bilberry, boneset, chamomile, dandelion, damiana, hawthorn, hops, hyssop, kava kava, lavender, lemongrass, motherwort, passionflower, skullcap, valerian, vervain

---

Appendicitis – *(inflammation of the appendix due to a blockage in the large intestine)*

Possible Factors – constipation, gastrointestinal infection, low-fiber diet, roundworm infestation

Common Symptoms – abdominal pain, coughing, deep breaths, diarrhea, fever, painful/bloody urine, sensitive to pain, sneezing

Helpful Nutrition – **Foods:** alfalfa sprouts, apples, apricots, artichokes, baked potatoes, beans, blueberries, bran, broccoli, cabbage, cantaloupe, carrots, cauliflower, corn, figs, fruits (organic), kelp, leafy green vegetables, lentils, oatmeal, pears, peas, raisins, salmon, soy foods, strawberries, whole grains; **Spices:** ginger; **Supplements:** (vitamins A, B-complex, C, E, zinc), aloe vera juice, echinacea, psyllium, wheatgrass juice; **Herbs:** slippery elm

---

Arteriosclerosis – *(hardening of the arteries resulting from a buildup of calcium deposits that increases the risk of hear attack and/or stroke)*

Possible Factors – aging, caffeine, diabetes, fatty/fried foods, heredity, high blood pressure & cholesterol, impaired circulation, inactivity, poor diet, smoking, stress, sugar, vitamin C deficiency, white flour

Common Symptoms – fatigue, high blood pressure, leg pain, numbness, sore muscles, weakness

Helpful Nutrition – **Foods:** almonds, apples, apricots, beans, beets, blueberries, bran, broccoli, cabbage, cantaloupe, carrots, cauliflower, celery, cranberry juice, figs, grapefruit juice, green tea (decaf), herring, kale, kelp, leafy green vegetables, legumes, mackerel, nuts/seeds (raw), oatmeal, olive oil, onions, pomegranates, potatoes (baked), salmon, soy foods, spinach, squash, sweet potatoes, tomatoes, tuna, wheat germ, whole grains; **Spices:** cayenne pepper, garlic, ginger, parsley, turmeric; **Supplements:** (vitamins A, B-complex, C, D & E, calcium, magnesium, selenium, zinc), aloe vera juice, apple cider vinegar, coconut oil, CoQ10, fish oil, flaxseed oil, ginkgo biloba, grape seed extract, royal jelly; **Herbs:** fenugreek, puncture vine, rose

Arthritis (osteo) – *(pain and inflammation of the joints caused by the deterioration of cartilage)*; (rheumatoid) – (*autoimmune disorder causing inflammation of tissues surrounding the joints)*

Possible Factors – aging, alcohol, bacterial/fungal/viral infections, caffeine, citrus fruits, dairy, excessive copper, iron or sodium, excessive uric acid, heredity, injury, nightshade vegetables (bell peppers, eggplant, paprika, tomatoes, white potatoes), obesity, poor diet, red meat, smoking, sugar, white flour

Common Symptoms – anemia, back pain/stiffness, bone crackling or popping sounds, bone spurs, breathing problems, fatigue, fever, inflammation, pain, redness, reduced range of motion, stiffness, swelling, tenderness, weight loss

Helpful Nutrition – **Foods:** alfalfa sprouts, almonds, apples, artichokes, asparagus, avocados, bananas, barley, beans (lima), beets, blueberries, broccoli, brown rice, Brussels sprouts, buckwheat, cabbage (green), canola oil, carrot juice, cauliflower, celery, cherries, chicken, eggs, grapes (red), halibut, herring, kale, kelp, leafy green vegetables, legumes, mackerel, mangoes, mangosteen, molasses, mushrooms (maitake, reishi), oats (raw), olive oil, onions, papayas, pears, peas, pineapples, plums, pomegranates, prunes, pumpkin seeds, rice bran, salmon, sardines, soy foods, strawberries, sweet potatoes, tuna, turkey, walnuts, watermelon, whole grains, wild rice, zucchini; **Spices:** basil, cayenne pepper, cilantro, cinnamon, dill, fennel, garlic, ginger, mustard, parsley, rosemary, sage, thyme, turmeric; **Supplements:** (vitamins A, B-complex, C, D, E & K, boron, calcium, germanium, magnesium, selenium, zinc), aloe vera juice, apple cider vinegar, chia seeds, chondroitin, coconut oil, fish oil, flaxseed oil, ginseng, glucosamine, grape seed extract, graviola, royal jelly, wheatgrass juice; **Herbs:** ashwagandha, bilberry, black cohosh, blessed thistle, boneset, bromelain, boldo, borage, boswellia, buchu, burdock, butcher's broom, calendula, cat's claw, chamomile, chanca peidra, chuchuhuasi, clove, cramp bark, dandelion, elder, eucalyptus, eyebright, feverfew, goldenseal, horse chestnut, horsetail, jatoba, juniper, licorice, macela, mullein, myrrh, nettle, olive leaf, Oregon grape, pau d'arco, pleurisy root, primrose, pygeum, sarsaparilla, white willow, wintergreen, yucca

---

Asthma – *(chronic lung disorder that narrows and constricts the airway)*

Possible Factors – adrenal disorders, anxiety, air pollution, allergies, anxiety, dairy, dust, dust mites, environmental toxins, excessive laughter, exercise, fear, feathers, food allergies, heredity, low blood sugar, mold, MSG, peanuts, processed foods, respiratory infection, secondhand smoke, smoking, stress, sugar, sulfites, white flour

Common Symptoms – inflammation of airway, difficulty breathing, chest tightness, coughing, wheezing

Helpful Nutrition – **Foods:** almonds, apples, bell peppers (orange), brown rice, buckwheat, cantaloupe, carrot juice, celery, cranberries, cucumber, eggplant, figs, grapefruit, grapes (red), green tea (decaf), honey (raw), kelp, leafy green vegetables, lemons, mushrooms (reishi), oats (raw), olive oil, onions, oranges, papayas, peaches, pears, pineapples, prunes, quinoa, sesame seeds, spinach, sweet potatoes, watermelon, whole grains, zucchini; **Spices:** basil, cayenne pepper, cinnamon, cumin, fennel, garlic, ginger, mustard, peppermint, rosemary, thyme, turmeric; **Supplements:** (vitamins A, B-complex, C, D, & E, calcium, magnesium, molybdenum, selenium, zinc), apple cider vinegar, CoQ10, cordyceps, echinacea, fish oil, flaxseed oil, ginkgo biloba, ginseng, grape seed extract, graviola, saw palmetto, wheatgrass juice; **Herbs:** chanca piedra, cramp bark, elder, eucalyptus, fenugreek, feverfew, goldenseal, hyssop, jatoba, juniper, licorice, macela, marshmallow, mullein, myrrh, nettle, primrose, passionflower, pau d'arco, pleurisy root, pygeum, red clover, slippery elm, tea tree, wild cherry

---

Atherosclerosis – *(hardening of the arteries from a buildup of fatty substances that increases the risk of hear attack and/or stroke)*

Possible Factors – aging, caffeine, diabetes, excessive sodium, fatty/fried foods, heredity, high blood pressure & cholesterol, impaired circulation, inactivity, poor diet, smoking, stress, sugar, white flour

Common Symptoms – fatigue, high blood pressure, leg pain, numbness, sore muscles, weakness

Helpful Nutrition – **Foods:** alfalfa sprouts, almonds, apples, bananas, barley, beets, berries, broccoli, brown rice, cabbage, carrots, cauliflower, celery, cranberry juice, grapefruit juice, grapes (red), green tea (decaf), herring, kale, kelp, leafy green vegetables, legumes, mackerel, mangoes, nuts/seeds (raw), oats (raw), olive oil, onions, papayas, pomegranates, prunes, quinoa, salmon, sardines, soy foods, spinach, sweet potatoes, tomatoes, tuna, watermelon, wheat germ, whole grains; **Spices:** cayenne pepper, garlic, ginger, mustard, parsley, sage, turmeric; **Supplements:** (vitamins A, B-complex, C, D & E, calcium, magnesium, selenium, zinc), aloe vera juice, apple cider vinegar, coconut oil, CoQ10, fish oil, flaxseed oil, grape seed extract, lecithin, milk thistle, royal jelly; **Herbs:** hawthorn, puncture vine

---

Benign Prostatic Hypertrophy (BPH) – *(enlarged prostate that may lead to prostate cancer)*

Possible Factors – alcohol, bacteria, caffeine, environmental toxins, heredity, hormone abnormality, kidney malfunction, poor diet

Common Symptoms – abdominal pain, bladder infection, bloody urine, difficulty urinating, fever, frequent and/or painful urination, kidney damage, pain after ejaculation, scrotum pain

Helpful Nutrition – **Foods:** apples (red), barley, beans, beets, bran, broccoli, brown rice, buckwheat, cabbage, carrot juice, celery, chicken, cranberries, cranberry juice, grapefruit, grapes (red), green tea (decaf), leafy green vegetables, lemons, limes, oatmeal, olive oil, onions, pomegranates, pumpkin seeds, quinoa, raisins, salmon, soy foods, tomato-based foods, turkey, watermelon, whole grains, zucchini; **Spices:** cayenne pepper, garlic, parsley, turmeric; **Supplements:** (vitamins A, B-complex, C & E, calcium, magnesium, selenium, zinc), acidophilus, echinacea, fish oil, flaxseed oil, ginseng, milk thistle, saw palmetto; **Herbs:** bilberry, buchu, corn silk, goldenseal, gravel root, hydrangea, jatoba, licorice, nettle, pau d'arco, pygeum, uva ursi

Bronchitis – *(inflammation and obstruction of the bronchial tubes in the lungs)*

Possible Factors – air pollution, allergies, ammonia, dairy, dust/fumes, emphysema, lung cancer, pneumonia, secondhand smoke, smoking, viral infection

Common Symptoms – difficulty breathing, chest pain, chills, coughing, foot/leg swelling, fever, headaches, lips appear bluish, mucus, runny nose, sore throat, wheezing

Helpful Nutrition – **Foods:** almonds, apples, bell peppers (orange), bran, brown rice, cantaloupe, carrot juice, celery, cranberries, cucumber, eggplant, figs, grapefruit, grapes (red), honey (raw), kelp, leafy green vegetables, lemons, limes, mushrooms (reishi), nuts/seeds (raw), olive oil, onions, oranges, papayas, peaches, pears, pineapples, prunes, quinoa, salmon, spinach, sweet potatoes, tomatoes, tuna, watermelon, whole grains; **Spices:** basil, cayenne pepper, cinnamon, cumin, fennel, garlic, ginger, mustard, peppermint, thyme, turmeric; **Supplements:** (vitamins A, B-complex, C & E, calcium, magnesium, zinc), aloe vera juice, apple cider vinegar, bromelain, CoQ10, cordyceps, echinacea, ginkgo biloba, ginseng, graviola, saw palmetto, wheatgrass juice; **Herbs:** boneset, chanca piedra, chickweed, chuchuhuasi, cramp bark, elder, eucalyptus, fenugreek, feverfew, goldenseal, hyssop, Irish moss, jaborandi, jatoba, juniper, licorice, marshmallow, mullein, myrrh, nettle, passionflower, pau d'arco, pygeum, red clover, slippery elm, tea tree, wild cherry, wormwood

---

Bulimia – *(binge-eating disorder characterized by self-induced purging or vomiting)*

Possible Factors – depression, junk food, low self esteem or self image, stress

Common Symptoms – excessive eating but no weight gain, hair loss, irregular heartbeat, lack of concentration, loss of fluid, low heart pulse, malnutrition, ulcers, vomiting, weakened immune system

Helpful Nutrition – **Foods:** apples, apricots, artichokes, baked potatoes, beans, blueberries, bran, broccoli, carrots, corn, figs, fruits (organic), granola, kelp, leafy green vegetables, lentils, oatmeal, pears, peas, raisins, salmon, soy foods, strawberries, sweet potatoes, whole grains; **Spices:** ginger; **Supplements:** (vitamins B-complex, C, E, calcium, potassium, selenium, zinc), acidophilus, fish oil, milk thistle, royal jelly; **Herbs:** licorice

---

Cancer (bladder) – *(cancer cells that develop in the tissues of the bladder)*

Possible Factors – aging, race (more common among Caucasians), caffeine, chemical exposure (hair dyes), chemotherapy, heredity, saccharin, sex (more common among men), smoking, urinary tract infection, postponing urination

Common Symptoms – abdominal/back pain, bloody/difficult/frequent/painful urination

Helpful Nutrition – **Foods:** apple sauce, bananas, beans, bell peppers (red), berries, broccoli, brown rice, Brussels sprouts, cabbage, carrots, cauliflower, celery, cottage cheese (low-fat), cranberries, grapefruit juice, kale, kelp, leafy green vegetables, lemons, limes, onions, oranges, pears, peaches, pineapples, pumpkin seeds, spinach, sweet potatoes, tomatoes, watermelon, whole grains; **Spices:** basil, cayenne pepper, cilantro, cinnamon, dill, garlic, ginger, oregano, parsley, sage, thyme, turmeric; **Supplements:** (vitamins A, B-complex, C & E, selenium, zinc), acidophilus, aloe vera juice, coconut oil, CoQ10, flaxseed oil, gingko biloba, milk thistle, wheatgrass juice; **Herbs:** buchu

---

Cancer (breast) – *(common form of cancer marked by an abnormal division of breast cells)*

Possible Factors – alcohol, environmental/industrial toxins, excessive estrogen, fatty or grilled foods, heredity, injury to the breast

Common Symptoms – lumps, yellow or bloody discharge from nipple

Helpful Nutrition – **Foods:** apples, avocados, barley, beets, berries, broccoli, brown rice, Brussels sprouts, buckwheat, cabbage, cantaloupe, carrots, cauliflower, celery, cherries, figs, grapefruit, grapes, green tea (decaf), kale, kelp, leafy green vegetables, lemons, limes, mangoes, mangosteen, millet, mushrooms (maitake), oats (raw), olive oil, onions, oranges, pineapples, plums, pomegranates, prunes, pumpkin seeds, quinoa, spinach, squash, sweet potatoes, tomatoes, watermelon, whole grains, yogurt; **Spices:** basil, cayenne pepper, cilantro, cumin, dill, fennel, garlic, mustard, oregano, parsley, rosemary, thyme, turmeric; **Supplements:** (vitamins A, B-complex, C, D & E, calcium, iodine, magnesium, potassium, selenium, zinc), acidophilus, aloe vera juice, brewer's yeast, CoQ10, echinacea, fish oil, flaxseed oil, ginkgo biloba, grape seed extract, graviola, milk thistle, psyllium, royal jelly, wheatgrass juice; **Herbs:** dandelion

---

Cancer (cervical) – *(cancer cells that develop in the cervix)*

Possible Factors – early sex & childbearing, infertility, multiple pregnancies (over 5), multiple sex partners, nutritional deficiencies, smoking, STD's (genital herpes, HIV, HPV), unprotected sex

Common Symptoms – bleeding after douching and/or sex, bleeding between menstrual periods, irregular discharge, heavy and/or long periods

Helpful Nutrition – **Foods:** apples, apricots, asparagus, avocados, barley, beef (lean), bell peppers (red & yellow), berries, bran, broccoli, brown rice, Brussels sprouts, buckwheat, cabbage, cantaloupe, carrots, celery, cheese, grapefruit, grapes (red), green tea, kale, kelp, leafy green vegetables, lemons, lentils, mangoes, mangosteen, millet, mushrooms (shiitake), nectarines, oats, olive oil, onions, orange juice, papayas, peaches, pears, pineapples, plums, pumpkin, quinoa, raisins, soy foods, spinach, sweet potatoes, strawberries, tomatoes, watermelon, whole grains, yogurt, zucchini; **Spices:** cayenne pepper, garlic, mustard, parsley, rosemary, thyme, turmeric; **Supplements:** (vitamins A, B-complex, C, D & E, calcium, selenium), acidophilus, aloe vera juice, apple cider vinegar, CoQ10, echinacea, fish oil, flaxseed oil, grape seed extract, graviola, milk thistle, wheatgrass juice; **Herbs:** astragalus

Cancer (colon) – *(tumor growth on the inner lining of the colon)*

Possible Factors – alcohol, calcium deficiency, constipation, grilled/charred foods, heredity, high-fat/low-fiber diet, obesity, red meat, white flour

Common Symptoms – abdominal pain, bloating, colitis, changes in color and/or consistency of stool, constipation, diarrhea, excessive cramps, fatigue, flatulence, rectal bleeding, sudden weight loss, weakness

Helpful Nutrition – **Foods:** almonds, apples, barley, beets, bell peppers (red), berries, bran, broccoli, brown rice, Brussels sprouts, buckwheat, cabbage, cantaloupe, carrots, cauliflower, celery, cherries, figs, grapefruit, grapes (red), green tea (decaf), kale, kelp, leafy green vegetables, leeks, lemons, mackerel, mangoes, mangosteen, millet, mustard greens, nectarines, oats (raw), olive oil, onions, papayas, peaches, pears, pineapples, plums, prunes, pumpkin seeds, quinoa, raisins, salmon, soy foods, spinach, squash, sweet potatoes, tomatoes, watermelon, wheat germ, whole grains, yogurt (low/non-fat), zucchini; **Spices:** basil, cayenne pepper, cilantro, cumin, fennel, garlic, mustard, oregano, parsley, rosemary, thyme, turmeric; **Supplements:** (vitamins A, B-complex, C, D & E, calcium, potassium, selenium, zinc), acidophilus, aloe vera juice, apple cider vinegar, CoQ10, cordyceps, echinacea, fish oil, flaxseed oil, grape seed extract, graviola, milk thistle, psyllium, wheatgrass juice; **Herbs:** astragalus, goldenseal, jaborandi, lemongrass, yellow dock

---

Cancer (esophageal) – *(cancer cells that develop in the middle to lower half of the esophagus)*

Possible Factors – aging, alcohol, environmental toxins, esophageal constriction, frequent heartburn, heredity, high-fat diet, pickled/salty foods, secondhand smoke, smoking, tylosis

Common Symptoms – difficulty swallowing, excessive mucus, vomiting, weight loss

Helpful Nutrition – **Foods:** amaranth, apples, barley, beans, beets, berries, broccoli, brown rice, Brussels sprouts, buckwheat, cabbage, carrot juice, celery, fruit juices (non-acidic), green tea (decaf), kale, kelp, leafy green vegetables, legumes, mangoes, millet, oat bran, onions, oranges, papayas, pasta, quinoa, tomatoes, salmon (broiled), soy foods, spinach, sweet potatoes, tomatoes, turkey (skinless), watermelon, whole grains; **Spices:** basil, garlic, oregano, parsley, turmeric; **Supplements:** (vitamins A, B-complex, C & E, calcium, molybdenum, selenium), aloe vera juice, coconut oil, CoQ10, fish oil, grape seed extract, graviola, spirulina, wheatgrass juice; **Herbs:** chamomile, dandelion

---

Cancer (laryngeal) – *(cancer cells that develop on the tissues of the larynx or voice box)*

Possible Factors – alcohol, environmental toxins (herbicides/pesticides), heredity, inhalation of fumes, secondhand smoke, smoking, vocal straining

Common Symptoms – bad breath, bloody saliva, frequent coughing, difficulty breathing/swallowing, earache, hoarseness, sore throat, weight loss

Helpful Nutrition – **Foods:** apple sauce, barley, beans, beets, berries, broccoli, brown rice, Brussels sprouts, buckwheat, cabbage, carrot juice, celery, figs, fruit juices (non-acidic), grapefruit, green tea (decaf), kale, kelp, leafy green vegetables, legumes, mangoes, millet, oat bran, onions, orange juice (diluted), papayas, pasta, pineapples, quinoa, tomatoes, salmon (broiled), soy foods, spinach, sweet potatoes, tomatoes, turkey (skinless), watermelon, whole grains; **Spices:** garlic, parsley, turmeric; **Supplements:** (vitamins A, B-complex, C & E, calcium, selenium), aloe vera juice, coconut oil, CoQ10, fish oil, grape seed extract, spirulina, wheatgrass juice; **Herbs:** dandelion

---

Cancer (lung) – *(common form of cancer that develops in the lung tissues)*

Possible Factors – air pollution, alcohol, asbestos, environmental toxins (herbicides/pesticides), heredity, secondhand smoke, smoking, tuberculosis, vitamin A deficiency

Common Symptoms – chest pain, chronic bronchitis, difficulty breathing, fatigue, fever, hoarseness, persistent coughing, phlegm with blood, swollen face/neck, weight loss, wheezing

Helpful Nutrition – **Foods:** apples, apricots, beans, beets, bell peppers (orange & red), berries, bran, broccoli, brown rice, Brussels sprouts, cabbage (red), cantaloupe, carrot juice, cauliflower, celery, cherries, grapefruit, grapes (red), green tea (decaf), kale, kiwi, leafy green vegetables, leeks, legumes, lemons, limes, mangoes, mangosteen, millet, mushrooms (shiitake), oats (raw), onions, oranges, papayas, peaches, pears, peas, pineapples, plums, pomegranates, pumpkin, quinoa, radish, salmon, soy foods, spinach, sunflower seeds, sweet potatoes, tangerines, tomatoes, watercress, watermelon, wheat germ, whole grains, wild rice, yogurt, zucchini; **Spices:** basil, cayenne pepper, fennel, garlic, mustard, oregano, parsley, rosemary, rye, thyme, turmeric; **Supplements:** (vitamins A, B-complex, C & E, calcium, potassium, selenium, zinc), acidophilus, aloe vera juice, brewer's yeast, coconut oil, CoQ10, cordyceps, echinacea, fish oil, flaxseed oil, grape seed extract, graviola, milk thistle, wheatgrass juice; **Herbs:** astragalus, pau d'arco, plantain, pleurisy root, slippery elm, wild cherry

---

Cancer (oral) – *(cancerous growth in the oral cavity or mouth)*

Possible Factors – alcohol, broken tooth, chewing tobacco, heredity, HPV virus, nutritional deficiencies, poor dental hygiene, smoking, ultraviolet light, weakened immune system

Common Symptoms – difficulty swallowing, discolored skin, mouth/tongue/throat sores, swollen jaw, toothache, voice changes, weight loss

Helpful Nutrition – **Foods:** amaranth, apple sauce, apricots, avocados, barley, beans, beets, berries, broccoli, brown rice, Brussels sprouts, buckwheat, cabbage, cantaloupe, carrot juice, celery, garlic, green tea (decaf), kale, kelp, leafy green vegetables, legumes, mangoes, millet, mushrooms, oat bran, onions, orange juice, papayas, pasta, pineapples, quinoa, tomatoes, salmon (broiled), soy foods, spinach, sweet potatoes, tomatoes, turkey (skinless), watermelon, whole grains; **Spices:** parsley, turmeric; **Supplements:** (vitamins A, B-complex, C & E, calcium, selenium), aloe vera juice, coconut oil, CoQ10, fish oil, grape seed extract, spirulina, wheatgrass juice; **Herbs:** dandelion

---

Cancer (ovarian) – *(cancer cells that develop in the tissues of the ovary)*

Possible Factors – asbestos, dairy, heredity, high-fat diet, not having children, obesity, radiation

Common Symptoms – bloated abdomen, constipation, diarrhea, frequent urination, vaginal bleeding

Helpful Nutrition – **Foods:** apples (red), bell peppers (red), berries, bran, broccoli, brown rice, Brussels sprouts, cabbage, carrots, cauliflower, celery, cranberry juice, grapefruit, grapes (red), green tea, kale, leafy green vegetables, lemons, mushrooms (shiitake), oats, olive oil, onions, peaches, pineapples, plums, prunes, pumpkin, raisins, salmon, spinach, sweet potatoes, tomatoes, watermelon, whole grains; **Spices:** basil, cayenne pepper, garlic, ginger, oregano, rosemary, parsley, turmeric; **Supplements:** (vitamins A, B-complex, C, E & K, calcium, potassium, selenium, zinc), acidophilus, aloe vera juice, CoQ10, echinacea, flaxseed oil, grape seed extract, wheatgrass juice; **Herbs:** astragalus

---

Cancer (pancreatic) – *(hard to detect cancer that develops from pancreatitis)*

Possible Factors – aging, fatty/fried/salty foods, heredity, obesity, pancreatitis, smoking

Common Symptoms – abdominal/back pain, depression, high blood pressure, jaundice, loss of appetite, muscle aches, nausea, sweating, vomiting, weight loss

Helpful Nutrition – **Foods:** almonds, bell peppers (red), blueberries, bran, brown rice, broccoli, Brussels sprouts, cabbage, canola oil, celery, cherries, chicken (skinless), cottage cheese, eggplant, grapes (red), green tea (decaf), kale, kelp, leafy green vegetables, mangoes, mushrooms (reishi), olive oil, onions, papayas, pomegranates, pumpkin seeds, salmon, soy foods, spinach, sweet potatoes, tomatoes, turkey (skinless), walnuts, whole grains, yogurt (non-fat), zucchini; **Spices:** basil, cayenne pepper, garlic, ginger, parsley, turmeric; **Supplements:** (vitamins A, B-complex, C & E, calcium, choline, chromium, inositol, magnesium, zinc), acidophilus, aloe vera juice, coconut oil, CoQ10, echinacea, fish oil, flaxseed oil, ginseng, grape seed extract, lecithin, milk thistle, royal jelly, wheatgrass juice; **Herbs:** boldo, burdock, dandelion, goldenseal, horsetail, mullein, red clover, uva ursi, wild cherry

---

Cancer (prostate) – *(cancer cells that develop in the prostate gland)*

Possible Factors – aging, carcinogens, excessive dairy, environmental toxins, excessive calcium, heredity, high-fat diet, lack of exercise, red meat

Common Symptoms – blood in the urine, burning sensation during urination, enlarged prostate, erectile or sexual dysfunction, frequent urination, inability to urinate, lower back pain

Helpful Nutrition – **Foods:** almonds, apples, apricots, avocados, barley, beans (garbanzo & kidney), beets, bell peppers (red), berries, broccoli, brown rice, Brussels sprouts, buckwheat, cabbage, carrots, cauliflower, celery, cranberry juice, figs, grapefruit, grapes (red), green tea (decaf), herring, kale, kelp, leafy green vegetables, lemons, limes, mackerel, mushrooms (maitake), oats bran, okra, olive oil, onions, oranges, papayas, peaches, pineapples, plums, pomegranates, prunes, pumpkin seeds, quinoa, raisins, salmon, sardines, sesame seeds, soy foods, spinach, squash, sweet potatoes, tomatoes, trout, walnuts, watercress, watermelon, whole grains, zucchini; **Spices:** basil, cayenne pepper, cilantro, fennel, garlic, oregano, parsley, peppermint, rosemary, thyme, turmeric; **Supplements:** (vitamins A, B-complex, C, D & E, magnesium, potassium, selenium, zinc), acidophilus, aloe vera juice, CoQ10, echinacea, fish oil, grape seed extract, graviola, milk thistle, saw palmetto, wheatgrass juice; **Herbs:** buchu, corn silk, goldenseal, gravel root, hydrangea, licorice, pau d'arco, pygeum

---

Cancer (skin) – *(malignant growth on the skin that forms primarily on sun-exposed areas of skin: face, scalp, neck, chest, lips, ears, nose and between the toes)*

Possible Factors – fair skin, heredity, industrial toxins, overexposure to sun, radiation exposure, smoking, tanning beds, weakened immune system

Common Symptoms – acute pain, bleeding, irregular-shaped moles, itching, large lumps, lesions, moles, overexposure to sun, skin discoloration, topical ulcers

Helpful Nutrition – **Foods:** almonds, berries, broccoli, Brussels sprouts, cabbage, canola oil, cauliflower, chives, fruit juices (organic), green tea (decaf), honey (raw), leafy green vegetables, lemons, limes, mackerel, onions, peaches, pumpkin seeds, salmon, soy foods, spinach, tomatoes, walnuts; **Spices:** basil, cayenne pepper, cilantro, garlic, mustard, oregano, parsley, rosemary, sage, thyme, turmeric; **Supplements:** (vitamins A, B-complex, C & E, calcium, potassium, selenium, zinc), acidophilus, aloe vera juice, coconut oil, CoQ10, echinacea, fish oil, flaxseed oil, grape seed extract, milk thistle, wheatgrass juice; **Herbs:** astragalus, birch, burdock, cat's claw, dandelion, echinacea, licorice, macela, olive leaf, pau d'arco, red clover

---

Cancer (stomach/gastric) – *(cancer cells that develop in the tissues lining the stomach)*

Possible Factors – aging, alcohol, anemia, heredity, low-fiber/high-fat diet, pickled foods, polyps, salty/smoked foods, smoking, stomach surgery

Common Symptoms – abdominal pain, bloating, bloody vomit, chronic heartburn, fatigue, weight loss

Helpful Nutrition – **Foods:** almonds, amaranth, apples, asparagus, barley, beans, beet juice, blueberries, broccoli, brown rice, buckwheat, cabbage, cantaloupe, carrot juice, celery, chicken (skinless), fruit juices (organic), grapefruit, green tea (decaf), kale, kelp, leafy green vegetables, legumes, mangoes, mangosteen, millet, oat bran, onions, oranges, papayas, pineapples, pumpkin, quinoa, raspberries, tomatoes, salmon (broiled), soy foods, spinach, squash, strawberries, sweet potatoes, tomatoes, tuna, turkey (skinless), vegetables (lightly steamed), watermelon, whole grains; **Spices:** basil, cilantro, garlic, oregano, parsley, turmeric; **Supplements:** (vitamins A, B-complex, C & E, calcium, selenium, zinc), acidophilus, aloe vera juice, chlorophyll, coconut oil, CoQ10, cordyceps, fish oil, grape seed extract, graviola, wheatgrass juice; **Herbs:** astragalus, birch, burdock, cat's claw, chamomile, chuchuhuasi, dandelion, echinacea, licorice, macela, olive leaf, pau d'arco, red clover

---

Cancer (testicular) – *(cancer cells that develop in the testicles)*

Possible Factors – alcohol, heredity, hernias, high-fat diet, lack of exercise, mumps

Common Symptoms – abdominal pain, blood in semen, bloody urine, breast enlargement, enlarged testicles or scrotum, lower back pain, lumps on testicle

Helpful Nutrition – **Foods:** almonds, apples, apricots, beets, bell peppers (red), berries, bran, broccoli, brown rice, Brussels sprouts, cabbage, cantaloupe, carrots, cauliflower, celery, cherries, grapes (red), green tea (decaf), leafy green vegetables, lemons, limes, mangoes, millet, mushrooms (reishi, shiitake), oat bran, onions, oranges, papayas, peaches, pineapples, plums, pumpkin, quinoa, salmon, soy foods, spinach, squash, sweet potatoes, tangerines, tomatoes, watermelon, whole grains, yogurt; **Spices:** basil, cayenne pepper, cilantro, fennel, garlic, oregano, parsley, rosemary, thyme, turmeric; **Supplements:** (vitamins A, B-complex, C & E, CoQ10, chromium, inositol, magnesium, potassium, selenium, zinc), acidophilus, aloe vera juice, fish oil, flaxseed oil, grape seed extract, graviola, milk thistle, saw palmetto, wheatgrass juice; **Herbs:** astragalus, birch, burdock, cat's claw, chaparral, chuchuhuasi, dandelion, echinacea, licorice, macela, olive leaf, pau d'arco, red clover

---

Canker Sores – *(small, inflamed ulcers of the mouth, gums, lips or tongue)*

Possible Factors – almonds, aspirin, cherries, chocolate, citrus fruits, coffee, gluten foods (barley, oats, rye, wheat), HIV, hormone imbalance, ibuprofen, nutritional deficiencies, peanuts, poor dental hygiene, spices, strawberries, stress, sugar, tomatoes, trauma, viral infections

Common Symptoms – blisters, burning or tingling sensation, mouth pain, reddened skin

Helpful Nutrition – **Foods:** broccoli, buttermilk, cabbage, cantaloupe, cottage cheese, kefir, legumes, onions (raw), papayas, potatoes, sweet potatoes, yogurt; **Spices:** garlic; **Supplements:** (vitamins A, B-complex, C & E, zinc), acidophilus, aloe vera juice, CoQ10, echinacea, fish oil, flaxseed oil, spirulina, wheatgrass juice; **Herbs:** burdock, calendula, lavender, myrrh, pau d'arco, red clover

Cardiovascular Disease (heart attack/stroke) – *(narrowing coronary arteries that obstruct sufficient amounts of blood and oxygen to the heart and brain)*

Possible Factors – air pollution, alcohol, arteriosclerosis/atherosclerosis, caffeine, diabetes, excessive sodium, fried foods, heredity, high blood pressure, kidney disease, lack of exercise, obesity, poor diet, red meat, smoking, stress, sugar, white flour

Common Symptoms – anxiety, chest pain, difficulty breathing and/or speaking, dizziness, ears ringing, fatigue, irregular heartbeat, skin discoloration, shortness of breath

Helpful Nutrition – **Foods:** alfalfa sprouts, almonds, apples, apricots, avocados, bananas, barley, beans, beets, bell peppers, berries, bran, broccoli, brown rice, buckwheat, cabbage, cantaloupe, carrots, cauliflower, celery, chicken (skinless), cranberry juice, figs, fish (broiled), grapefruit, grapes (red), green tea, halibut, kale, kelp, leafy green vegetables, lemons, limes, mackerel, mangoes, mangosteen, mineral water w/ lemon, mushrooms (maitake, reishi, shiitake), oats (raw), olive oil, onions, oranges, papayas, peaches, pineapples, pomegranates, prunes, quinoa, salmon, sardines, soy foods, spinach, sweet potatoes, tomatoes, trout, tuna, turkey (skinless), watermelon, whole grains, zucchini; **Spices:** basil, cayenne pepper, cumin, dill, fennel, garlic, ginger, mustard, parsley, peppermint, rosemary, sage, turmeric; **Supplements:** (vitamins A, B-complex, C & E, calcium, choline, magnesium, potassium, selenium, silicon, vanadium, zinc), acidophilus, aloe vera juice, apple cider vinegar, chia seeds, coconut oil, CoQ10, cordyceps, echinacea, fish oil, flaxseed oil, ginkgo biloba, grape seed extract, graviola, psyllium, wheatgrass juice; **Herbs:** ashwagandha, black cohosh, borage, chanca peidra, hawthorn, horse chestnut, horsetail, kudzu, motherwort, pau d'arco, uva ursi, wood betony

---

Carpal Tunnel Syndrome (CTS) – *(repetitive motion disorder mainly affecting the wrists, hands and fingers as well as the legs, back and neck)*

Possible Factors – alcohol, arthritis, bone spurs, diabetes, excessive sodium, gout, heredity, hormonal changes, hypothyroidism, injuries, obesity, pregnancy, repetitive motion, water retention

Common Symptoms – burning/tingling sensation, impaired coordination, numbness, soreness

Helpful Nutrition – **Foods:** almonds, asparagus, avocados, bananas, beets, broccoli, brown rice, cabbage, chicken, eggs, kelp, olive oil, onions, papayas, pineapples, rhubarb, salmon, soy foods, spinach, sweet potatoes, tuna, whole grains; **Spices:** cayenne pepper, cumin, garlic, ginger, parsley, sage, turmeric; **Supplements:** (vitamins A, B-complex, C & E, calcium, manganese, potassium, selenium, zinc), acidophilus, aloe vera juice, bromelain, CoQ10, fish oil, flaxseed oil, ginkgo biloba, grape seed extract, St. John's wort, wheatgrass juice; **Herbs:** butcher's broom, chamomile, corn silk, marshmallow, nettle

Cataracts – *(opaque clouding of the eye lens that adversely affects vision)*

Possible Factors – aging, dehydration, deterioration of lens fiber, diabetes, environmental toxins, eye injuries, heredity, high blood pressure, metal toxicity, MSG, overexposure to sun, poor diet, radiation, smoking, stagnation of lens fluid

Common Symptoms – blurry/cloudy vision, difficulty reading, double vision, loss of vision, light/glare sensitivity, poor night vision

Helpful Nutrition – **Foods:** apricots, bananas, bell peppers (orange), berries, broccoli, cabbage, cantaloupe, carrots, cauliflower, figs, fruit juices (organic), grapefruit, green tea (decaf), kale, leafy green vegetables, nuts/seeds (raw), onions, papayas, peaches, pineapples, prunes, pumpkin seeds, quinoa, raisins, salmon, soy foods, spinach, squash, sweet potatoes, tomatoes, watercress, watermelon, zucchini; **Spices:** cayenne pepper, garlic; **Supplements:** (vitamins A, B-complex, C & E, calcium, manganese, selenium, zinc), acidophilus, apple cider vinegar, CoQ10, fish oil, flaxseed oil, ginkgo biloba, grape seed extract; **Herbs:** bayberry, eyebright, fenugreek

---

Celiac Disease – *(digestive disorder where the lining of the small intestine is damaged by gluten)*

Possible Factors – gluten foods (barely, oats, rye, wheat products: bulgur, durum, farro, kamut, spelt; related grains: bran, couscous, malt, matzo, miso and semolina), heredity, pregnancy, stress, surgery

Common Symptoms – abdominal pain, anemia, bloating, bruising, depression, diarrhea, fatigue, flatulence, hair loss, headache, heartburn, infertility, irritability, nausea, nosebleeds, rashes, seizures, vitamin B12 and K deficiency, vomiting, weight loss

Helpful Nutrition – **Foods:** alfalfa sprouts, almonds, amaranth, apples, artichokes, avocados, basmati rice, beans (garbanzo, kidney, lima), blackberries, broccoli, brown rice, cabbage, cantaloupe, carrots, celery, chicken (skinless), corn, eggs, figs, green tea (decaf), kelp, leafy green vegetables, lentils, mangoes, melons, millet, molasses, olive oil, onions, papayas, pears, peas, pomegranates, potatoes, pumpkin seeds, prunes, quinoa, raisins, raspberries, salmon, soy flour, spinach, strawberries, sweet potatoes, sunflower seeds, tomatoes, wild rice, yogurt (gluten-free); **Spices:** cayenne pepper, cilantro, garlic, ginger, peppermint, thyme; **Supplements:** (vitamins A, B-complex, C, D, E & K, calcium, chromium, copper, magnesium, zinc), acidophilus, aloe vera juice, bentonite, coconut oil, CoQ10, flaxseed oil, grape seed extract, milk thistle, psyllium, spirulina; **Herbs:** burdock, dandelion, horsetail, kudzu, olive leaf, primrose, slippery elm

---

Chickenpox – *(highly contagious Varicella-zoster virus (VZV) common among children under 12)*

Possible Factors – airborne transmission, direct physical contact, droplet contact (sneezing, coughing)

Common Symptoms – blisters, fever, headache, itching, low appetite, rashes, red spots, shingles

Helpful Nutrition – **Foods:** alfalfa sprouts, almonds, artichokes, bananas, barley, beans (kidney), beets, bell peppers, broccoli, brown rice, cabbage, carrot juice, cauliflower, distilled water w/ lemon, figs, fruit juices (organic), grapefruit, green tea (decaf), kale, kelp, leafy green vegetables, lemons, mangoes, melons, molasses, mushrooms (maitake, reishi), olive oil, onions, papayas, peas, prunes, raisins, rice bran, soy foods, spinach, tomatoes, walnuts, wheat bran, whole grains; **Spices:** cayenne pepper, fennel, garlic, ginger, parsley, rosemary, thyme, turmeric; **Supplements:** (vitamins A, B-complex, C, D, E & K, calcium, choline, inositol, magnesium, molybdenum, selenium, zinc), acidophilus, aloe vera juice, bentonite, brewer's yeast, coconut oil, CoQ10, cordyceps, echinacea, flaxseed oil, grape seed extract, grapefruit seed extract, graviola, lecithin, milk thistle, royal jelly, wheatgrass juice; **Herbs:** acerola, barberry, blessed thistle, boldo, burdock, chicory, corn silk, dandelion, gentian, goldenseal, horsetail, Oregon grape, puncture vine, red clover, rose, sarsaparilla, vervain, wormwood

---

Cirrhosis – *(hardening of liver cells and scarring of tissues that causes irreversible liver damage)*

Possible Factors – alcohol, blood transfusions, excessive vitamin A, hepatitis, high-fat diet, viral infections

Common Symptoms – constipation, diarrhea, fatigue, fever, inflamed liver, poor appetite, red palms, upset stomach, vomiting, weight loss

Helpful Nutrition – **Foods:** alfalfa sprouts, almonds, artichokes, bananas, barley, beans (kidney), beets, bell peppers, broccoli, brown rice, cabbage, carrot juice, cauliflower, distilled water w/ lemon, figs, grapefruit, green tea (decaf), kale, kelp, leafy green vegetables, lemons, mangoes, melons, molasses, mushrooms (maitake, reishi), olive oil, onions, papayas, peas, prunes, raisins, rice bran, soy foods, spinach, tomatoes, walnuts, wheat bran, whole grains; **Spices:** cayenne pepper, fennel, garlic, ginger, parsley, rosemary, thyme, turmeric; **Supplements:** (vitamins A, B-complex, C, D, E & K, calcium, choline, inositol, magnesium, molybdenum, selenium, zinc), acidophilus, aloe vera juice, bentonite, brewer's yeast, chia seeds, coconut oil, CoQ10, cordyceps, echinacea, flaxseed oil, grape seed extract, graviola, lecithin, milk thistle, royal jelly, wheatgrass juice; **Herbs:** acerola, barberry, blessed thistle, boldo, boswellia, burdock, chicory, corn silk, dandelion, gentian, goldenseal, gotu kola, horsetail, licorice, Oregon grape, puncture vine, red clover, rose, sarsaparilla, vervain, wormwood, yellow dock

---

Colitis (ulcerative) – *(inflamed colon tissues that develop ulcers)*

Possible Factors – alcohol, antibiotics, bacterial/viral infection, dairy, food allergies, heredity, poor diet, spices, stress, weakened immune system

Common Symptoms – abdominal/back/neck pain, bloating, bloody/mucus diarrhea, cramping, dehydration, fatigue, fever, flatulence, frequent bowel movements, hardened stools, inflammation, night sweats, weight loss

Helpful Nutrition – **Foods:** (*avoid raw vegetables/foods - only baked, boiled, broiled or steamed) apples (peeled), applesauce, artichokes, bananas, cabbage juice, carrot juice, cauliflower, chicken (skinless), eggs, green tea (decaf), leafy green vegetables, lentils, onions, papayas, pears, pineapples, pomegranates, potatoes (skinless), salmon, soy foods, sweet potatoes, turkey (skinless), vegetable juice; **Spices:** fennel, garlic, ginger, turmeric; **Supplements:** (vitamins A, B-complex, C, E & K, calcium, iron, magnesium, selenium, zinc), acidophilus, aloe vera juice, apple cider vinegar, bromelain, coconut oil, CoQ10, fish oil, grape seed extract, milk thistle, psyllium, wheatgrass juice; **Herbs:** boswellia, buchu, burdock, chamomile, dandelion, kudzu, nettle, pau d'arco, red clover, slippery elm

---

Common Cold – *(upper respiratory viral infection)*

Possible Factors – viral infections, weakened immune system

Common Symptoms – bronchitis, congestion, coughing, fatigue, fever, headaches, runny nose, sinus infection, sneezing, sore throat, watery eyes, weakened immune system

Helpful Nutrition – **Foods:** almonds, broths, celery, chicken soup, green tea (decaf), leafy green vegetables, mangoes, mushrooms (reishi, shiitake), onions, papayas, pineapples, pomegranates, soy foods, turkey; **Spices:** cayenne pepper, cilantro, cumin, garlic, ginger, mustard, peppermint, sage, thyme, turmeric; **Supplements:** (vitamins A, C, selenium, zinc), acidophilus, apple cider vinegar, bromelain, chia seeds, CoQ10, echinacea, ginseng, grape seed extract, grapefruit seed extract, graviola, milk thistle, wheatgrass juice; **Herbs:** boneset, chamomile, chanca piedra, chickweed, elder, eucalyptus, feverfew, gentian, goldenseal, jaborandi, kudzu, lavender, macela, myrrh, nettle, pau d'arco, pleurisy root, sangre de grado, slippery elm, tea tree, vervain, white oak, white willow, wild cherry, wintergreen, wormwood, yohimbe

---

Constipation – *(difficult or infrequent bowel movements)*

Possible Factors – aging, alcohol, antidepressants, dairy, dehydration, diabetes, excessive calcium, excessive meat consumption, insufficient fiber and/or fluids, iron supplements, lack of exercise, muscle disorders, poor diet, salt, soft drinks, sugar, white flour

Common Symptoms – bad breath, body odor, colitis, decreased absorption of nutrients, digestive disorders, fatigue, flatulence, headaches, hemorrhoids, hernia, insomnia, obesity, varicose veins

Helpful Nutrition – **Foods:** alfalfa sprouts, almonds, apples, apple juice, apricots, avocados, asparagus, bananas, barley, beans, beets, bell pepper, blackberries, bran, broccoli, brown rice, Brussels sprouts, buckwheat, cabbage, carrots, cauliflower, celery, cranberries, coconut, dates, figs, grapes, honey (raw), kale, leafy green vegetables, limes, molasses, nuts/seeds (raw), oats (raw), okra, olive oil, papayas, peaches, pears, peas, prune juice, pumpkin seeds, raisins, sauerkraut, spinach, sweet potatoes, sunflower seeds, whole grains, yogurt, zucchini; **Spices:** basil, cayenne pepper, cilantro, cinnamon, dill, fennel, garlic, ginger, parsley, peppermint, rosemary; **Supplements:** (vitamins A, B-complex, C & E, selenium, zinc), acidophilus, aloe vera juice, apple cider vinegar, bentonite, brewer's yeast, coconut oil, CoQ10, flaxseed oil, grape seed extract, milk thistle, psyllium, wheatgrass juice; **Herbs:** acerola, chicory, dandelion, elder, kudzu, slippery elm, wintergreen, yerba mate

---

Crohn's Disease – *(inflammatory bowel disorder of the small intestine and/or the digestive tract)*

Possible Factors – colitis, heredity, nutritional deficiencies, weakened immune system

Common Symptoms – abdominal pain, bloody diarrhea, fatigue, fevers, flatulence, heredity, inflammation, infrequent bowel movements, loss of appetite, ulcers, vomiting, weight loss

Helpful Nutrition – **Foods:** (*avoid raw vegetables/foods - only baked, boiled, broiled or steamed) artichokes, broccoli, Brussels sprouts, cabbage juice, carrots, cauliflower, celery, chicken (skinless), distilled water w/ lemon, green tea (decaf), kale, kelp, leafy green vegetables, lentils, mangoes, mangosteen, papayas, peaches, pineapples, pomegranates, salmon, spinach, sweet potatoes, tofu, tomatoes; **Spices:** cilantro, cinnamon, dill, fennel, garlic, ginger, peppermint, turmeric; **Supplements:** (vitamins A, B-complex, C, D, E & K, calcium, magnesium, potassium, selenium, zinc), acidophilus, aloe vera juice, bentonite, bromelain, coconut oil, CoQ10, echinacea, flaxseed oil, fish oil, graviola, milk thistle, wheatgrass juice; **Herbs:** burdock, chamomile, fenugreek, licorice, macela, marshmallow, pau d'arco, red clover, rose, slippery elm, yerba mate

---

Cystic Fibrosis – *(inherited disease causing a progressive decline of the lungs, liver, pancreas, sinuses and digestive system)*

Possible Factors – heredity, mutation in the CFTR gene

Common Symptoms – bacterial infection in the lungs, chest tightness, coughing, difficulty breathing, enlarged fingers, profuse sweating, thick mucus, wheezing

Helpful Nutrition – **Foods:** alfalfa sprouts, apricots, avocadoes, bell peppers, broccoli, brown rice, carrots, cauliflower, celery, figs, green tea (decaf), honey (raw), kelp, leafy green vegetables, mushrooms (shiitake), nuts/seeds (raw), olive oil, onions, papayas, pineapples, pumpkin, spinach, squash, sweet potatoes; **Spices:** cayenne pepper, garlic, ginger, peppermint, thyme, turmeric; **Supplements:** (vitamins A, B-complex, C, E & K, calcium, germanium, iron, selenium, zinc), acidophilus, aloe vera juice, bromelain, CoQ10, flaxseed oil, grape seed extract, milk thistle, psyllium, wheatgrass juice; **Herbs:** boswellia, hyssop, licorice, mullein, nettle

---

Depression – *(psychiatric disorder that diminishes mental and physical health)*

Possible Factors – alcohol, artificial sweeteners, caffeine, chemical or nutritional imbalance, family and/or relationship problems, food allergies, heredity, hypoglycemia, lack of exercise, loss of a loved one, negative thinking, poor diet, social inadequacy, stress, sugar, trauma, wheat products, white flour

Common Symptoms – backaches, bipolar disorder, chronic pain, difficulty concentrating or thinking, digestive disorders, fatigue, feeling helpless, feelings of worthlessness, headaches, insomnia, loss of appetite, loss of interest, low moods and self esteem, oversleeping, restlessness, social withdrawal, suicidal thoughts, weight loss or weight gain

Helpful Nutrition – **Foods:** apples, apricots, bananas, barley, bran, broccoli, brown rice, cabbage, chicken, leafy green vegetables, legumes, mackerel, millet, nuts/seeds (raw), oats (raw), olive oil, onions, salmon, soy foods, tuna, turkey, whole grains, yogurt; **Spices:** cayenne pepper, fennel, garlic, ginger, peppermint, rosemary; **Supplements:** (vitamins A, B-complex, C, calcium, choline, chromium, inositol, magnesium, selenium, zinc), acidophilus, aloe vera juice, apple cider vinegar, fish oil, flaxseed oil, ginkgo biloba, ginseng, graviola, milk thistle, royal jelly, St. John's wort, wheatgrass juice; **Herbs:** gotu kola, kava kava, lavender, licorice, oat straw, vervain

---

Dermatitis (eczema) – *(chronic skin disorder causing inflammation of the skin)*

Possible Factors – allergies, cosmetics, dry skin, food allergies (dairy, eggs, peanuts, soy foods, wheat products), heredity, latex, low levels of stomach acid, metal toxicity, ointments, perfumes, poisons, poor diet, stress, sugar, weakened immune system, white flour

Common Symptoms – blisters, flaky/scaly skin, hay fever, itching, leathery skin, psoriasis, rashes, red inflamed skin, scratching, skin discoloration & tenderness, swelling

Helpful Nutrition – **Foods:** brown rice, leafy green vegetables, millet, olive oil, onions, peaches, pineapples, pomegranates, salmon; **Spices:** garlic; **Supplements:** (vitamins A, B-complex, C, & E, zinc), aloe vera juice, apple cider vinegar, brewer's yeast, bromelain, coconut oil, CoQ10, fish oil, flaxseed oil, ginkgo biloba, grape seed extract, graviola, psyllium, royal jelly, wheatgrass juice; **Herbs:** borage, chamomile, chickweed, comfrey (topically), dandelion, goldenseal (topically), gotu kola, Irish moss, lavender, lemongrass, marshmallow, nettle, oat straw, olive leaf, Oregon grape, pau d'arco, primrose, sangre de grado, tea tree oil (topically), wormwood, yellow dock

---

Diabetes (Type 2) – *(pancreas produces low levels of insulin causing high blood-sugar levels)*

Possible Factors – chromium deficiency, dried fruits, excessive sodium/sugar, heredity, hypothyroidism, lack of exercise, obesity, pancreas malfunction, saturated fats, smoking, viral infections, white flour

Common Symptoms – blurred vision, confusion, disorientation, dizziness, excessive sweating, excessive urination, extreme thirst, heart and kidney disease, high blood pressure, hunger, mouth infections, nerve damage, numbness, slow metabolism

Helpful Nutrition – **Foods:** almonds, amaranth, apples, artichokes, asparagus, avocados, barley, berries, beans (except fava), bell peppers, broccoli, brown rice, Brussels sprouts, buckwheat, cabbage, cantaloupe, carrots (with meals), cauliflower, celery, cheese, cherries, corn, cucumber, eggplant, egg yolks, figs, grapefruit, green tea (decaf), kelp, leafy green vegetables, leeks, legumes, mangoes, millet, mushrooms (maitake, reishi), oat bran, olive oil, onions (red), organic vegetable juices, papayas, peanuts, pears, plums, pomegranates, prunes, pumpkin seeds, quinoa, radishes, salmon, sesame seeds, soy foods, spinach, sprouts, sweet potatoes, sunflower seeds, tomatoes, walnuts, whole grains, yogurt (non-fat), zucchini; **Spices:** basil, cayenne pepper, cilantro, cinnamon, garlic, ginger, mustard; **Supplements:** (vitamins A, B-complex, C, E & K, calcium, chromium, inositol, magnesium, manganese, potassium, vanadium, zinc), acidophilus, aloe vera juice, apple cider vinegar, bentonite, chia seeds, CoQ10, cordyceps, flaxseed oil, fish oil, ginseng, grape seed extract, milk thistle, psyllium, royal jelly, spirulina, wheatgrass juice; **Herbs:** astragalus, bilberry, buchu, dandelion, eucalyptus, fenugreek, kudzu, red clover, uva ursi

---

Diarrhea – *(digestive disorder marked by frequent, loose stools)*

Possible Factors – alcohol, antibiotics, apple juice, artificial sweeteners, bacterial or viral infection, caffeine, cold liquids, colitis, contaminated water, Crohn's disease, fatty/fried/spicy foods, food allergies (dairy, eggs, peanuts, soy foods, wheat products), intestinal parasites, pancreas malfunction, stress

Common Symptoms – abdominal pain, blood in stool, cramping, dehydration, fever, loose/watery stools, loss of salts and electrolytes, thirst, vomiting

Helpful Nutrition – **Foods:** amaranth, applesauce, artichokes, bananas, blueberries, brown rice, carob flour, carrot juice, celery, honey (raw), kelp, leafy green vegetables, olive oil, potatoes, pumpkin, radishes, rice flour, toast, tomatoes; **Spices:** cayenne pepper, cinnamon, fennel, garlic, ginger, oregano, peppermint, sage, turmeric; **Supplements:** (vitamins A, B-complex, C, E & K, calcium, potassium, zinc), acidophilus, apple cider vinegar, bentonite, flaxseed oil, ginseng, grapefruit seed extract, grape seed extract, psyllium, St. John's wort; **Herbs:** acerola, astragalus, barberry, boneset, boswellia, chamomile, chuchuhuasi, fenugreek, feverfew, goldenseal, kudzu, marshmallow, meadowsweet, olive leaf, pleurisy root, rose, slippery elm, white oak, wild cherry

---

Diverticulitis – *(infection and inflammation of the diverticula)*

Possible Factors – aging, alcohol, chills, heredity, low-fiber diet, obesity, pain, smoking, stress

Common Symptoms – abdominal pain on left side, bloating, bloody stool, constipation or diarrhea, cramping, dehydration, fever, flatulence, inflammation, nausea

Helpful Nutrition – **Foods:** alfalfa sprouts, apples, apricots, asparagus, bananas, beans (green), beets, bell peppers, berries, bran, brown rice, cantaloupe, carrot juice, celery, cherries, chicken (skinless), cucumber, dates, eggs, figs, kelp, mangoes, mushrooms, nectarines, oat bran, olive oil, onions, oranges, papayas, peaches, pears, peas, salmon, soy foods, spinach, squash, sweet potatoes, watermelon, zucchini; **Spices:** cayenne pepper, garlic, ginger, oregano, thyme, turmeric; **Supplements:** (vitamins A, B-complex, C, E & K, calcium, sulfur, zinc), acidophilus, aloe vera juice, flaxseed oil, psyllium, wheatgrass juice; **Herbs:** chamomile, goldenseal, pau d'arco, red clover, slippery elm

---

Ear Infection – *(bacterial or viral infection that inflames the ear canal)*

Possible Factors – allergenic foods (dairy, fruits, peanut butter, sugar, wheat), cold temperatures, high altitudes, upper respiratory infection

Common Symptoms – coughing, diarrhea, difficulty hearing, dizziness, ear discharge, fever, inflamed ear canal, ringing in the ears, sore throat, throbbing/painful ear, vomiting

Helpful Nutrition – **Foods:** leafy green vegetables, olive oil, onions, salmon; **Spices:** garlic; **Supplements:** (vitamins A, B-complex, C, & E, manganese, zinc), CoQ10, echinacea, flaxseed oil, grape seed extract, grapefruit seed extract, wheatgrass juice; **Herbs:** goldenseal, mullein

---

Edema (fluid retention) – *(swelling caused by excessive accumulation of water in the body's tissues)*

Possible Factors – AIDS/HIV, allergies, arthritis, blood pressure medication, burns, cirrhosis, congestive heart failure, diabetes, excessive sodium/sugar, lack of exercise, ibuprofen, kidney disorders, lymphatic malfunction, PMS, pregnancy, protein deficiency, thyroid malfunction, vein damage

Common Symptoms – bloated abdomen, body aches, chest pain, difficulty breathing, joint stiffness, stretched skin, swollen/puffy skin, rapid weight gain

Helpful Nutrition – **Foods:** alfalfa sprouts, apple juice, artichokes, asparagus, bananas, beets, bell peppers, broccoli, brown rice, Brussels sprouts, cabbage, cantaloupe, carrots, celery, chicken (skinless), cottage cheese (low-fat), cranberry juice, cucumber, eggs, fish (broiled), fruits (organic), grapes (red), green tea (decaf), horseradish, kelp, molasses, onions, pineapples, potatoes, spinach, sunflower seeds, tomatoes, turkey (skinless), walnuts, watermelon, wheat germ, yogurt (non-fat); **Spices:** garlic, parsley, turmeric; **Supplements:** (vitamins B-complex, C, D & E, calcium, magnesium, manganese, potassium), brewer's yeast, bromelain, CoQ10; **Herbs:** buchu, burdock, butcher's broom, corn silk, dandelion, gotu kola, gravel root, jaborandi, marshmallow, uva ursi

---

Emphysema – *(chronic lung disorder caused by long-term smoking and/or exposure to air pollution)*

Possible Factors – heredity, industrial toxins, poor air quality, secondhand smoke, smoking

Common Symptoms – coughing, difficulty breathing, dizziness, fatigue, headaches, phlegm, vision impairment, wheezing

Helpful Nutrition – **Foods:** alfalfa sprouts, almonds, apples, apricots, asparagus, avocados, berries, brown rice, carrot juice, celery, chicken (skinless), grapes (red), kale, kelp, leafy green vegetables, lemons, limes, millet, olive oil, onions, oranges, papayas, peaches, pears, pineapples, plums, pumpkin seeds, salmon, soy foods, spinach, sunflower seeds, tomatoes, turkey (skinless), watercress, whole grains; **Spices:** basil, cayenne pepper, cinnamon, cumin, fennel, garlic, ginger, mustard, rosemary, thyme, turmeric; **Supplements:** (vitamins A, B-complex, C & E, calcium, copper, magnesium, zinc), chlorophyll, CoQ10, cordyceps, fish oil, flaxseed oil, ginkgo biloba, wheatgrass juice; **Herbs:** astragalus, licorice, fenugreek, mullein

---

Epilepsy – *(neurological disorder characterized by unprovoked, recurring seizures)*

Possible Factors – air pollution, alcohol, allergies, aluminum toxicity, artificial sweeteners, caffeine, drug withdrawal, fever, flashing/flickering lights, fried foods, hunger, infections, insomnia, low blood sugar, nutritional deficiencies, sage, smoking, stress, sugar, trauma, white flour

Common Symptoms – chewing motion, difficulty breathing, fatigue, hearing sounds, lack of muscle tone, memory loss, seizures, temporary loss of consciousness, unaware of surroundings, wheezing

Helpful Nutrition – **Foods:** alfalfa sprouts, asparagus, beans (green), beet juice, broccoli, carrot juice, cauliflower, celery, cherries, chicken (skinless), cucumber, grapes (red), leafy green vegetables, olive oil, peas, salmon, spinach, yogurt; **Spices:** cayenne pepper, garlic, turmeric; **Supplements:** (vitamins A, B-complex, C, calcium, magnesium, selenium, zinc), acidophilus, coconut oil, fish oil, flaxseed oil; **Herbs:** black cohosh, blue cohosh, chamomile, hyssop, macela

---

Fatigue – *(debilitating disorder characterized by an extreme lack of energy)*

Possible Factors – age, allergies, anemia, arthritis, depression, fungal/viral infections, heredity, hormonal imbalance, hypothyroidism, low blood pressure, low blood sugar, metal toxicity, weakened immune system

Common Symptoms – anxiety, candidiasis, difficulty concentrating, fatigue, fever, headache, insomnia, jaundice, loss of appetite, memory loss, mood swings, muscle spasms, nasal congestion, night sweats, respiratory infections, sensitivity to light, sore muscles, sore throat

Helpful Nutrition – **Foods:** alfalfa sprouts, almonds, bananas, bell peppers, bran, broccoli, brown rice, buckwheat, cabbage, cantaloupe, carrots, figs, fruit juices (organic), grapes (red), green tea (decaf), honey (raw), leafy green vegetables, mangoes, mangosteen, melons, molasses, mushrooms (maitake, reishi, shiitake), oats (raw), onions, papayas, pineapples, prunes, pumpkin seeds, quinoa, raisins, spinach, tofu, tomatoes, walnuts, watermelon, whole grains; **Spices:** cayenne pepper, fennel, garlic, ginger, thyme, turmeric; **Supplements:** (vitamins A, B-complex, C & E, calcium, choline, cobalt, iodine, magnesium, manganese, phosphorus, potassium, selenium, zinc), acidophilus, aloe vera juice, apple cider vinegar, brewer's yeast, chia seeds, coconut oil, CoQ10, cordyceps, echinacea, ginkgo biloba, ginseng, grape seed extract, grapefruit seed extract, graviola, milk thistle, psyllium, royal jelly, spirulina, wheatgrass juice; **Herbs:** astragalus, dandelion, gotu kola, guarana, jatoba, licorice, maca, olive leaf, Oregon grape, skullcap

---

Fever – *(abnormal increase in body temperature)*

Possible Factors – antibiotics, bacterial/viral infections, extreme sunburn, heat exhaustion, stress, weakened immune system

Common Symptoms – chills/coldness, coughing, dehydration, elevated heart rate, fatigue, headaches, irregular heartbeat, loss of appetite, muscle aches, shivering, sore throat

Helpful Nutrition – **Foods:** broth, celery juice, fruit juices (organic), soups; **Spices:** garlic, ginger, oregano, sage, thyme, turmeric; **Supplements:** (vitamins A, B-complex, C, selenium), coconut oil, echinacea, graviola, royal jelly, vervain, wheatgrass juice; **Herbs:** acerola, barberry, bayberry, boneset, borage, calendula, chamomile, chuchuhuasi, elder, eucalyptus, fenugreek, feverfew, gentian, hyssop, jaborandi, lemongrass, myrrh, nettle, olive leaf, pau d'arco, pleurisy root, white oak, white willow, wormwood, yerba buena, yohimbe

---

Fibromyalgia – *(autoimmune disorder marked by widespread chronic muscle pain)*

Possible Factors – immune system malfunction, heredity, nightshade vegetables (bell peppers, eggplant, tomatoes, white potatoes)

Common Symptoms – anxiety, burning sensation, dizziness, dry eyes and mouth, fatigue, food allergies, headaches, impaired coordination, insomnia, irregular heartbeat, memory loss, muscle pain, PMS, throbbing, stiffness

Helpful Nutrition – **Foods:** brown rice, celery juice, chicken (skinless), kelp, leafy green vegetables, millet, mushroom (reishi), nuts/seeds (raw), olive oil, soy foods, turkey (skinless); **Spices:** cayenne pepper, garlic, ginger, rosemary, turmeric; **Supplements:** (vitamins A, B-complex, C, D & E, calcium, chromium, magnesium, manganese, selenium, zinc), acidophilus, aloe vera juice, apple cider vinegar, coconut oil, CoQ10, echinacea, flaxseed oil, ginkgo biloba, grape seed extract, lecithin, milk thistle, royal jelly, wheatgrass juice; **Herbs:** astragalus, boswellia, burdock, dandelion, kava kava, licorice, pau d'arco, red clover, skullcap, valerian

---

Flatulence – *(excessive gas produced in the digestive tract)*

Possible Factors – aging, bacterial infection, caffeine, cruciferous vegetables (broccoli, Brussels sprouts, cabbage, cauliflower, radishes), food allergies, gallbladder disorders, gas-forming foods (apples, apricots, bagels, bananas, beans, beer, bran, breads, brown rice, carrots, celery, cucumber, dairy, dried fruits, eggplant, leeks, onions, potatoes, pretzels, prunes, raisins, soft drinks), indigestion, nutritional deficiencies, pancreas malfunction, poor diet, spicy foods, sugar, white flour

Common Symptoms – foul odor, insomnia, irregular heartbeat, memory loss, muscle pain, nausea, PMS, throbbing, stiffness

Helpful Nutrition – **Foods:** alfalfa sprouts, bell peppers, grapes, green tea (decaf), lemons, mangoes, papayas, peanut butter, pumpkin, soy foods, yogurt; **Spices:** basil, cayenne pepper, cilantro, dill, ginger, oregano, peppermint tea, rosemary, thyme, turmeric; **Supplements:** (vitamins A, B-complex, C, calcium, magnesium, manganese, selenium, zinc), acidophilus, CoQ10, flaxseed oil, ginkgo biloba, grape seed extract, wheatgrass juice; **Herbs:** anise, astragalus, clove, kudzu, lemongrass, yerba buena

---

Food Poisoning – *(illness contracted through the consumption of bacteria, viruses, parasites or toxins: botulism, E. coli, rotavirus, salmonella, staph infection)*

Possible Factors – contaminated/spoiled foods, raw fish, unclean cooking surfaces, undercooked meats

Common Symptoms – abdominal/back/neck pain, bloating, diarrhea, cramping, dehydration, fatigue, fever, flatulence, frequent bowel movements, headaches, night sweats, weight loss, vomiting

Helpful Nutrition – **Foods:** distilled water w/lemon, fruits and vegetables (raw), kelp, lemon juice, pomegranates, whole grains; **Spices:** cayenne pepper, cilantro, cinnamon, garlic, ginger, turmeric; **Supplements:** (vitamins C & E, potassium), acidophilus, apple cider vinegar, coconut oil, grapefruit seed extract, milk thistle; **Herbs:** goldenseal, red clover

---

Gallbladder Disorders (gallstones) – *(crystalline stone formations caused by elevated levels of bile and cholesterol in the gallbladder)*

Possible Factors – animal fats, bile tract disorders, blood disorders, cirrhosis, excessive dairy, fried/spicy foods, heredity, lack of exercise, margarine, obesity, oxalate-rich foods, sugar, white flour

Common Symptoms – abdominal and chest pain, chills, fever, inflamed gallbladder, jaundice, nausea, radiating pain in back and shoulders, vomiting

Helpful Nutrition – **Foods:** alfalfa sprouts, almonds, apples, applesauce, apricots, artichokes, barley, beets, beet juice, cottage cheese (low-fat), eggs, kelp, lemons, mangoes, olive oil, papayas, peaches, pears, quinoa, soy foods, yogurt (low-fat); **Spices:** fennel, garlic, ginger, oregano, parsley, peppermint, sage, turmeric; **Supplements:** (vitamins A, B-complex, C, D & E, calcium, choline, magnesium, manganese, selenium, zinc), acidophilus, aloe vera juice, apple cider vinegar, coconut oil, CoQ10, flaxseed oil, ginkgo biloba, grape seed extract, lecithin, milk thistle; **Herbs:** barberry, boldo, burdock, cascara sagrada, chanca peidra, cramp bark, dandelion, vervain, white oak, wormwood

Gingivitis (periodontal disease) – *(inflammatory disorder affecting the gums and teeth)*

Possible Factors – blood disease, heredity, poor brushing habits, poor diet, sugar, tooth grinding, vitamin and mineral deficiency

Common Symptoms – abscesses, bad breath, bloody gums, loose/missing teeth, mouth/tooth pain, oral inflammation, red/soft gums

Helpful Nutrition – **Foods:** broccoli, brown rice, cabbage, carrot juice, cauliflower, celery, collard greens, green tea (decaf), kale, legumes, melons, mushrooms, onions, pumpkin, quinoa, raisins, salmon, soy foods, spinach, whole grains; **Spices:** cayenne pepper, garlic, ginger, peppermint, sage, turmeric; **Supplements:** (vitamins A, B-complex, C & E, calcium, iron, magnesium, zinc), aloe vera juice, coconut oil, CoQ10, ginseng, grape seed extract, wheatgrass juice; **Herbs:** chamomile, horsetail, myrrh

---

Glaucoma – *(optical nerve damage caused by elevated fluid pressure in the eyes)*

Possible Factors – aging, alcohol, African ancestry, caffeine, diabetes, eye problems, heredity, high blood pressure, nutritional deficiencies, prolonged computer or TV usage, smoking, steroids, stress

Common Symptoms – blindness, blurred vision, eye pain, headaches, light sensitivity, loss of peripheral vision, nausea, seeing halos of light, vision impairment, vomiting

Helpful Nutrition – **Foods:** berries, broccoli, cabbage, cantaloupe, carrots, cauliflower, collard greens, grapes (red), green tea (decaf), leafy green vegetables, mangoes, onions, papayas, quinoa, salmon, soy foods, spinach, squash, sweet potatoes, watercress; **Spices:** cayenne pepper, garlic; **Supplements:** (vitamins A, B-complex, C & E, calcium, choline, inositol, magnesium, selenium, zinc), CoQ10, flaxseed oil, ginkgo biloba; **Herbs:** bilberry, chickweed, eyebright, rose

---

Gout – *(acute form of arthritis causing pain and inflammation of the big toe)*

Possible Factors – abnormal kidney function, alcohol, antibiotics, aspirin, caffeine, dehydration, diabetes, excessive uric acid, fried foods, heredity, high blood pressure, inactivity, leukemia, lymphoma, nightshade vegetables (bell peppers, eggplant, tomatoes, white potatoes), obesity, organ meats, red meat, smoking, stress, sugar, white flour

Common Symptoms – acute pain of the big toe (also ankles, elbows, knees, wrists), chills/fever, inflammation/pain at night, kidney stones, limited movement, reddish swollen skin

Helpful Nutrition – **Foods:** alfalfa sprouts, almonds, avocados, bananas, beans, beets, blueberries, broccoli, brown rice, cabbage, cantaloupe, carrots, celery, cherries, grapes (red), kale, kelp, leafy green vegetables, mangoes, mangosteen, millet, nuts/seeds (except peanuts), olive oil, onions, papayas, peas, pineapples, plums, pomegranates, quinoa, soy foods, squash, strawberries, sweet potatoes, walnuts, whole grains; **Spices:** cayenne pepper, garlic, ginger, parsley, turmeric; **Supplements:** (vitamins A, B-complex, C & E, calcium, chromium, magnesium, potassium, selenium, zinc), aloe vera juice, apple cider vinegar, chondroitin, coconut oil, CoQ10, fish oil, flaxseed oil, ginkgo biloba, glucosamine, grape seed extract, milk thistle, royal jelly, wheatgrass juice; **Herbs:** bilberry, birch, boldo, boswellia, burdock, butcher's broom, burdock, dandelion, hyssop, juniper, lemongrass, sarsaparilla, yucca

---

Halitosis (chronic bad breath) – *(excessive protein and toxin buildup in the mouth and digestive tract)*

Possible Factors – alcohol, bronchitis, cirrhosis, coffee, constipation, diabetes, digestive disorders, fasting, fever, gingivitis, metal toxicity, poor dental hygiene, poor diet, respiratory tract infection, sinusitis, smoking, spices, stress, sugar

Common Symptoms – unpleasant breath odor

Helpful Nutrition – **Foods:** apples, avocadoes, beets, cantaloupe, carrots, celery, cucumber, grapefruit, green tea, leafy green vegetables, kale, lemons, oranges, pineapples, pomegranates, rice milk, spinach, sunflower seeds (after meals), tomatoes, watercress, yogurt; **Spices:** basil, ginger, parsley, peppermint, rosemary, thyme, turmeric; **Supplements:** (vitamins A, B-complex & C, zinc), acidophilus, wheatgrass juice; **Herbs:** barberry, fenugreek, myrrh, tea tree oil mouthwash, yerba buena

---

Headache – *(excessive tension causing recurring or severe head pain)*

Possible Factors – alcohol, allergies, anxiety, aspartame, caffeine, chewing gum, coffee, constipation, dehydration, excessive sun exposure, eye strain, food allergies (dairy, eggs, peanuts, soy foods, wheat products), high blood pressure, hormone imbalance, hunger, lack of oxygen, MSG, muscle tension, nitrates, nutritional deficiencies, perfumes, poor circulation, sinus pressure, stress, sugar, sulfites

Common Symptoms – blurred/impaired vision, dizziness, fatigue, insomnia, irritability, lack of concentration, loss of appetite, sensitivity to light or noise, throbbing pain

Helpful Nutrition – **Foods:** bran, broccoli, brown rice, celery, leafy green vegetables, quinoa, salmon, spinach, whole grains; **Spices:** cayenne pepper, cinnamon, garlic, ginger, parsley, peppermint, rosemary, sage, thyme, turmeric; **Supplements:** (vitamins A, B-complex, C & E, calcium, magnesium, potassium, zinc), apple cider vinegar, bromelain, CoQ10, fish oil, flaxseed oil, ginkgo biloba, milk thistle; **Herbs:** acerola, burdock, chamomile, fenugreek, feverfew, guarana, kava kava, kudzu, lavender, lemongrass, marshmallow, meadowsweet, motherwort, skullcap, wood betony, wormwood, yerba buena, yucca

<u>Heartburn</u> (<u>acid reflux</u>) – *(stomach acid backs up in the esophagus causing a burning sensation and pain in the chest and stomach)*

<u>Possible Factors</u> – alcohol, aspirin, caffeine, cheese, chocolate, citrus fruits (acidic), coffee, fatty/fried/spicy foods, gravies, ibuprofen, lying down/sleeping on right side of body, raw onions, peppermint, smoking, soft drinks, tomato-based foods, stress, sugar, white flour

<u>Common Symptoms</u> – bloating, burping, difficulty swallowing, esophageal burning/cancer, flatulence, hoarseness, insomnia, nausea, shortness of breath, sore throat

<u>Helpful Nutrition</u> – **Foods:** apples, apricots, bananas, cabbage juice, celery, leafy green vegetables, mangoes, papayas, pears, pineapples, potato juice (raw), soy foods, watermelon, yogurt (non-fat); **Spices:** dill, fennel, ginger, turmeric; **Supplements:** (vitamin B-complex, calcium, magnesium, potassium), acidophilus, aloe vera juice, apple cider vinegar, bromelain, flaxseed oil, grape seed extract, milk thistle; **Herbs:** chamomile, dandelion, goldenseal, marshmallow, meadowsweet, plantain, slippery elm, white willow, wood betony, yerba mate

---

<u>Hemophilia</u> (<u>poor blood clotting</u>) – *(inability of blood to coagulate and form clots due to insufficient blood proteins)*

<u>Possible Factors</u> – chromosome abnormality, heredity

<u>Common Symptoms</u> – bloody urine, internal bleeding, nervous system bleeding, pain/swelling in joints and muscles, spontaneous bleeding, warm prickly sensation

<u>Helpful Nutrition</u> – **Foods:** alfalfa sprouts, asparagus, beet greens, broccoli, Brussels sprouts, cabbage, cauliflower, celery, collard greens, cucumber, egg yolks, green tea (decaf), kale, leafy green vegetables, liver, mustard greens, okra, peas, spinach, turnip greens; **Spices:** cayenne pepper, parsley; **Supplements:** (vitamins B-complex, C & K, calcium, magnesium, phosphorus), aloe vera juice, grape seed extract, wheatgrass juice; **Herbs:** bilberry, hawthorn, nettle

---

<u>Hemorrhoids</u> – *(enlarged, swollen veins around the anus and colon)*

<u>Possible Factors</u> – alcohol abuse, coffee, constipation, food allergies, heavy lifting, inactivity, insufficient dietary fiber, obesity, poor diet, pregnancy, red meat, spicy foods, standing/sitting for too long, straining during bowel movement

<u>Common Symptoms</u> – burning sensation, inflammation, itching, rectal bleeding, seepage, swelling

<u>Helpful Nutrition</u> – **Foods:** alfalfa sprouts, apples, apricots, bananas, barley, beans (green, lima), beets,

berries (red), Brazil nuts, broccoli, brown rice, Brussels sprouts, bok choy, cabbage, carrots, cauliflower, celery, distilled water w/ lemon, kale, kelp, leafy green vegetables, mangoes, mangosteen, molasses, oat bran, oranges, papayas, peaches, pears, peas, pineapples, plums, pomegranate juice, salmon, sesame seeds, spinach, strawberries, sweet potatoes, Swiss chard, tangerines, tofu, turkey, whole grains; **Spices:** cayenne pepper, dill, fennel, garlic, parsley, turmeric; **Supplements:** (vitamins A, B-complex, C, D, E & K, calcium, choline, inositol, iron, magnesium, potassium), acidophilus, aloe vera gel (topically), aloe vera juice, apple cider vinegar, coconut oil, CoQ10, fish oil, flaxseed oil, psyllium; **Herbs:** butcher's broom, comfrey, goldenseal, pau d'arco, plantain, slippery elm, white oak

---

Hepatitis (A, B & C) – *(viral infection causing inflammation of the liver)*

(hepatitis A) – *(causes acute liver disease, easily spread, liver can heal within a few months)*
(hepatitis B) – *(spread through contact with infected blood, most recover, 15% develop cirrhosis)*
(hepatitis C) – *(most serious, progressive damage to liver, usually leads to chronic liver disease)*

Possible Factors – alcohol, autoimmune disorders, blood transfusions, body piercings/tattoos, environmental toxins, fatty/fried foods, fecal contamination, heredity, metabolism disorders, non-steroidal anti-inflammatory drugs (ibuprofen, naproxen), raw fish, sharing needles (IV drug use), shellfish, unprotected sex, viral infections, water contamination

Common Symptoms – abdominal pain, drowsiness, fever, headaches, lack of bile production, loss of appetite, muscle and joint pain, nausea, skin discoloration, vomiting, weakness

Helpful Nutrition – Foods: apples, artichokes, asparagus, avocados, barley, beans, beets, blueberries, broccoli, brown rice, cabbage, carrot juice, cauliflower, celery, cucumber, figs, grapefruit, green tea (decaf), kale, leafy green vegetables, lemons, mushrooms (maitake, reishi, shiitake), olive oil, onions, spinach, squash, sweet potatoes, whole grains; Spices: cayenne pepper, fennel, garlic, ginger, parsley, thyme, turmeric; Supplements: (vitamins A, B-complex, C, E & K, calcium, choline, inositol, magnesium, molybdenum, selenium), aloe vera juice, coconut oil, CoQ10, cordyceps, flaxseed oil, grape seed extract, lecithin, milk thistle, psyllium, royal jelly, wheatgrass juice; Herbs: acerola, barberry, blessed thistle, boldo, boswellia, burdock, cascara sagrada, chicory, corn silk, dandelion, gentian, goldenseal, gotu kola, licorice, Oregon grape, puncture vine, red clover, sarsaparilla, vervain, wormwood, yellow dock

---

Herpes – *(highly contagious herpes simplex virus usually associated with sexually transmitted diseases)*

Possible Factors – indirect contact (sharing clothing, drinking glasses, towels, soap), direct physical contact, sharing a bed, oral sex, unprotected sex

Common Symptoms – blindness, burning sensation, cold sores, fatigue, fever, groin pain, itching, multiple sclerosis, painful urination, shingles, skin irritation, weakened immune system

Helpful Nutrition – **Foods:** almonds, barley, cashews, cheese, chicken (skinless), corn, dairy, eggs, grapefruit, leafy green vegetables, mushrooms (reishi, shiitake), nuts/seeds (raw), oats (raw), pomegranates, potatoes, quinoa, salmon, soy foods, whole grains, yogurt; **Spices:** cayenne pepper, garlic, sage; **Supplements:** (vitamins A, B-complex, C & E, calcium, magnesium, zinc), brewer's yeast, coconut oil, CoQ10, echinacea, fish oil, flaxseed oil, grapefruit seed extract, graviola, milk thistle, spirulina, St John's wort; **Herbs:** astragalus, black walnut (topically), goldenseal, licorice, olive leaf, red clover, sangre de grado, tea tree oil (topically)

High Cholesterol – *(excessive levels of cholesterol in the blood which may cause clogged arteries)*

Possible Factors – aging, alcohol, animal fats, coffee, fried foods, heredity, inactivity, lack of sunlight, obesity, oral contraceptives, red meat, smoking, vitamin C deficiency

Common Symptoms – arteriosclerosis/atherosclerosis, bruising, chest pain, cold extremities, confusion, dizziness, fatigue, lack of coordination, nausea, numbness, vision problems, vomiting

Helpful Nutrition – **Foods:** alfalfa sprouts, almonds, apples, apricots, avocados, bananas, barley, beans, beets, bell peppers, berries (except cherries), broccoli, brown rice, buckwheat, cabbage, cantaloupe, carrots, cauliflower, celery, cottage cheese (low-fat), figs, grapefruit, grapes (red), green tea (decaf), honey (raw), kale, kelp, leafy green vegetables, lentils, lemons, limes, mangoes, mushrooms (maitake, reishi, shiitake), oat bran, olive oil, onions, oranges, papayas, peaches, pomegranates, prunes, pumpkin seeds, quinoa, salmon, soy foods, spinach, tomatoes, tuna, turkey, walnuts, watermelon, whole grains, yogurt, zucchini; **Spices:** basil, cayenne pepper, cilantro, cinnamon, dill, fennel, garlic, ginger, mustard, oregano, parsley, rosemary, sage, thyme, turmeric; **Supplements:** (vitamins A, B-complex, C & E, calcium, choline, germanium, inositol, selenium, vanadium), aloe vera juice, apple cider vinegar, brewer's yeast, chia seeds, coconut oil, CoQ10, cordyceps, fish oil, flaxseed oil, ginseng, grape seed extract, graviola, lecithin, milk thistle, psyllium, royal jelly, spirulina, wheatgrass juice; **Herbs:** black cohosh, black walnut, boswellia, dandelion, fenugreek, hawthorn, hyssop, kudzu, lemongrass, oat straw, olive leaf, puncture vine, red clover, valerian

---

Hypertension (high blood pressure) – *(systemic arterial blood pressure is abnormally elevated)*

Possible Factors – aging, alcohol, animal fats, artificial sweeteners, caffeine, calcium deficiency, fried foods, heart or nervous system problems, ibuprofen, obesity, red meat, smoking, sodium, stress, sugar

Common Symptoms – chest pain, irregular heartbeat, kidney failure, morning headaches, nausea, vision problems, vomiting

Helpful Nutrition – **Foods:** alfalfa sprouts, almonds, apples, apricots, asparagus, bananas, barley, beans, beets, bell peppers, berries (except cherries), broccoli, brown rice, buckwheat, cabbage, cantaloupe, carrots, cauliflower, celery, chicken, eggplant, figs, grapefruit, grapes (red), green tea (decaf), kale, kelp, leafy green vegetables, lemons, limes, mangoes, melons, millet, mushrooms (maitake, reishi, shiitake), oat bran, olive oil, onions, oranges, papayas, peaches, peas, pineapples, pomegranates, prunes, pumpkin seeds, quinoa, raisins, salmon, sesame seeds, soy foods, spinach, sweet potatoes, tomatoes, turkey, watermelon, whole grains, zucchini; **Spices:** basil, cayenne pepper, cinnamon, dill, fennel, garlic, oregano, parsley, rosemary, thyme, turmeric; **Supplements:** (vitamins A, B-complex, C, & E, calcium, choline, germanium, inositol, magnesium, potassium, selenium, vanadium, zinc), aloe vera juice, apple cider vinegar, bromelain, chia seeds, coconut oil, CoQ10, cordyceps, fish oil, flaxseed oil, ginkgo biloba, grape seed extract, graviola, lecithin, psyllium, spirulina, wheatgrass juice; **Herbs:** black cohosh, boswellia, chamomile, dandelion, fenugreek, hawthorn, hyssop, kudzu, nettle, oat straw, olive leaf, passionflower, pau d'arco, primrose, puncture vine, valerian

---

Hyperthyroidism (Graves' disease) – *(thyroid gland produces excessive amounts of thyroid hormone)*

Possible Factors – immune system malfunction, inflamed thyroid, nicotine patches, pituitary tumor, thyroid tumor, smoking, stress

Common Symptoms – anxiety, breathlessness, decreased menstruation, depression, diarrhea, fatigue, feeling 'hot', high blood pressure, increased bowel movements, increased metabolism, insomnia, loss of libido, lumps/tumors, nausea, poor nutrient absorption, rapid heartbeat, sweating, tremors, vomiting, weakness, weight loss

Helpful Nutrition – **Foods:** bell peppers, blueberries, broccoli, Brussels sprouts, cabbage, cauliflower, cereals, cherries, chicken, eggs, kale, leafy green vegetables, mangoes, olive oil, onions, papayas, peaches, pears, salmon, spinach, squash, tomatoes, turnips, whole grains; **Spices:** cayenne pepper, ginger, turmeric; **Supplements:** (vitamins B-complex, C & E, calcium, phosphorus, zinc), brewer's yeast, CoQ10, fish oil, flaxseed oil, milk thistle

---

Hypoglycemia (low blood sugar) – *(low levels of glucose in the blood)*

Possible Factors – adrenal fatigue, alcohol, caffeine, heredity, kidney disease, lack of exercise, large meals, pancreatitis, poor diet, red meats, smoking, stress, thyroid or pituitary malfunction, white flour

Common Symptoms – anxiety, blurred vision, chest pain, confusion, cravings for sweets, decreased menstruation, depression, diarrhea, dizziness, eye pain, fatigue, headache, hunger, insomnia, irregular heartbeat, mood swings, nausea, rapid heartbeat, seizures, sweating, swollen feet, tremors, weakness

Helpful Nutrition – **Foods:** almond butter, apples, apricots, artichokes, avocados, bananas, beans (except fava), bran, broccoli, brown rice, cantaloupe, carrots, chicken (skinless), cottage cheese (low-fat), grapefruit, kefir, lemons, lentils, molasses, mushrooms (maitake), nuts/seeds (raw), oat bran, peaches, peanut butter, pears, plums, potatoes, salmon, spinach, squash, sweet potatoes, tofu, turkey (skinless); **Spices:** cayenne pepper, garlic, parsley; **Supplements:** (vitamins B-complex, C, & E, calcium, chromium, magnesium, manganese, sulfur, zinc), brewer's yeast, echinacea, milk thistle, psyllium, spirulina, wheatgrass juice; **Herbs:** dandelion, gentian, pau d'arco, uva ursi

Hypotension (low blood pressure) – *(insufficient blood flowing through the arteries and veins)*

Possible Factors – Addison's disease, allergic reactions, blood clot in lungs, dehydration, diarrhea, diabetes, excessive exercise, fever, heat exhaustion, liver disease, loss of blood, medications, nutritional deficiencies, pancreatitis, pregnancy, thyroid malfunction, weak heart

Common Symptoms – acidosis, chest pain, dizziness, fainting, fatigue, headache, heart attack, major organ damage or failure, nausea, stroke, thirst, vomiting

Helpful Nutrition – **Foods:** alfalfa sprouts, apples, apricots, bananas, beetroot juice, berries, broccoli, brown rice, Brussels sprouts, cabbage, carrots, cauliflower, cantaloupe, chicken (skinless), fruit juices (organic), green tea, kelp, leafy green vegetables, low-carb foods, nuts/seeds (raw), olive oil, salmon, soy foods, whole grains; **Spices:** cayenne pepper, cinnamon, ginger, parsley, rosemary, turmeric; **Supplements:** (vitamins B-complex & C, iron, potassium, selenium, zinc), flaxseed oil, ginseng, wheatgrass juice; **Herbs:** ashwagandha, hawthorn, motherwort

---

Hypothyroidism – *(thyroid gland produces insufficient amounts of thyroid hormone)*

Possible Factors – caffeine, Hashimoto's disease, excessive sodium, sugar, tap water, white flour

Common Symptoms – coldness, coma (after illness/trauma), confusion, constipation, depression, dry hair, fatigue, fertility issues, hair loss, hoarseness, loss of appetite, migraines, muscle cramps and weakness, premenstrual pain, respiratory infections, scaly/discolored skin, slowed heart rate, weight gain

Helpful Nutrition – **Foods:** alfalfa sprouts, apricots, avocadoes, bananas, barley, beans (lima), bok choy, cauliflower, cheese, chicken (skinless), corn, dates, egg yolks, kelp, mangoes, molasses, oatmeal, papayas, parsley, peas, potatoes, prunes, salmon, seeds (raw), strawberries, sweet potatoes, whole grains; **Spices:** cayenne pepper; **Supplements:** (vitamins A, B-complex, C, & E, iodine, iron, selenium, zinc), acidophilus, brewer's yeast, coconut oil, fish oil, St. John's wort; **Herbs:** bayberry, black cohosh, gentian, goldenseal, primrose

---

Impotence (erectile dysfunction) – *(inability for men to achieve or sustain an erection)*

Possible Factors – aging, alcohol, atherosclerosis, dairy, diabetes, high blood pressure, hormone malfunction, junk food, lack of exercise, medications, metal toxicity, obesity, smoking, STD's, stress

Common Symptoms – depression, inability to achieve or sustain an erection, loss of libido

Helpful Nutrition – **Foods:** almonds, baked potatoes, beans, brown rice, chicken (skinless), kelp, mackerel, nuts/seeds (raw), oatmeal, oysters, pomegranate juice, pumpkin seeds, salmon, sardines, soy foods, spinach, sweet potatoes, tuna, turkey, watermelon, whole grains; **Spices:** cayenne pepper, garlic, turmeric; **Supplements:** (vitamins A, B-complex, C, & E, iodine, molybdenum, selenium, zinc), cordyceps, fish oil, ginkgo biloba, ginseng, milk thistle, royal jelly, saw palmetto; **Herbs:** ashwagandha, dong quai, gotu kola, hydrangea, primrose, pygeum, sarsaparilla, yohimbe

---

Indigestion – *(uncomfortable feeling in the stomach due to excessive acid levels)*

Possible Factors – acidic foods (beans, bell peppers, chocolate, citrus fruits, coffee, pasta, red meat, tomatoes), alcohol, caffeine, dairy, obesity, pickled/spicy foods, poor diet, soft drinks, sugar, white flour

Common Symptoms – abdominal pain, allergies, burping, bloating, constipation, diarrhea, fatigue, flatulence, heartburn, insomnia, muscle pain, nausea, skin disorders, vomiting, weight loss

Helpful Nutrition – **Foods:** alfalfa sprouts, almonds, apricots, artichokes, brown rice, buckwheat, figs, kale, mangoes, olive oil, papayas, peaches, pineapples, pomegranates; **Spices:** basil, cinnamon, cumin, dill, fennel, ginger, mustard, oregano, parsley, rosemary, sage; **Supplements:** (vitamins B-complex and K, manganese, selenium, zinc), acidophilus, aloe vera juice, apple cider vinegar, bentonite, coconut oil, flaxseed oil, ginseng, grapefruit seed extract, graviola, lecithin, milk thistle, wheatgrass juice; **Herbs:** astragalus, barberry, buchu, burdock, chamomile, chicory, dandelion, goldenseal, horsetail, Irish moss, kava kava, kudzu, lemongrass, meadowsweet, passionflower, red clover, slippery elm, white willow, wild cherry, yerba buena, yerba mate

---

Infertility – *(Women: failure to conceive or carry a pregnancy, Men: abnormal sperm cell production)*

Possible Factors – age, blocked fallopian tubes, caffeine, lack of progesterone, medications, ovulatory impairment, radiation, smoking, STD's

Common Symptoms – failure to conceive or carry a pregnancy

Helpful Nutrition – **Foods:** alfalfa sprouts, barley, beets, broccoli, Brussels sprouts, cabbage, carrots, cauliflower, collard greens, figs, kale, kelp, onions, oysters, pumpkin seeds, salmon, sweet potatoes, tofu, walnuts, whole grains; **Spices:** cayenne pepper, fennel, turmeric; **Supplements:** (vitamins A, B-complex, C & E, calcium, iron, manganese, selenium, zinc), aloe vera juice, CoQ10, cordyceps, fish oil, flaxseed oil, ginseng, grape seed extract, milk thistle, royal jelly, saw palmetto, wheatgrass juice; **Herbs:** black cohosh, damiana, maca, primrose, sarsaparilla, valerian

---

Inflammation – *(reaction to allergies, illness or injury that causes swelling, redness and pain)*

Possible Factors – alcohol, allergies, arthritis, asthma, bacterial infection, citrus fruits, colitis, Crohn's disease, dairy, drug abuse, excessive uric acid, menopause, nutritional deficiencies, vegetable oils, red meat, stress, sugar, toxins, trauma, ulcers, white flour

Common Symptoms – headaches, muscle stiffness, redness, swollen joints, warm sensation, worn cartilage

Helpful Nutrition – **Foods:** alfalfa sprouts, almonds, apples, artichokes, beets, blueberries, broccoli, brown rice, buckwheat, cabbage, canola oil, cauliflower, celery, grapes (red), green tea (decaf), halibut, herring, kale, kelp, lentils, mackerel, mangoes, mangosteen, mushrooms (maitake, reishi), olive oil, onions, papayas, peaches, pineapples, pomegranates, prunes, pumpkin seeds, salmon, spinach, strawberries, sweet potatoes, tuna, turkey (skinless), walnuts, watermelon, whole grains; **Spices:** basil, cayenne pepper, cilantro, cinnamon, dill, fennel, garlic, ginger, mustard, parsley, peppermint, rosemary, sage, thyme, turmeric; **Supplements:** (vitamins A, B-complex, C & E, calcium, choline, selenium, zinc), acidophilus, aloe vera juice, apple cider vinegar, bromelain, chlorophyll, coconut oil, CoQ10, fish oil, flaxseed oil, ginkgo biloba, ginseng, goldenseal, grape seed extract, royal jelly, saw palmetto, wheatgrass juice; **Herbs:** ashwagandha, bilberry, birch, black cohosh, blessed thistle, boldo, boneset, borage, boswellia, buchu, butcher's broom, calendula, cat's claw, chamomile, chanca peidra, chuchuhuasi, clove, cramp bark, dandelion, elder, eucalyptus, eyebright, feverfew, horse chestnut, jatoba, juniper, licorice, macela, mullein, myrrh, nettle, olive leaf, Oregon grape, pau d'arco, pleurisy root, primrose, pygeum, red clover, white willow, wintergreen, yellow dock, yucca

---

Influenza (flu) – *(highly contagious influenza A or B virus affecting the respiratory system)*

Possible Factors – airborne transmission, person-to-person contact, droplet contact (sneezing, coughing)

Common Symptoms – asthma, body ache, coughing, diarrhea, dry throat, fatigue, fever, headache, hot/cold sweats, inner ear infection, nausea, painful eyes, pneumonia, runny nose, sneezing, sore throat, vomiting, weak immune system

Helpful Nutrition – **Foods:** apples, avocados, berries, fruit juices (organic), grapefruit, herbal teas, leafy green vegetables, legumes, lemons, limes, mushrooms (maitake, reishi, shiitake), nuts/seeds (raw), orange juice, pears, pomegranates, soups/broths, sugar-free foods, tomatoes, vegetable juices (beet, celery, watercress), whole grains; **Spices:** cayenne pepper, garlic, ginger, parsley, peppermint, sage, thyme, turmeric; **Supplements:** (vitamins A, B-complex, C, D & E, iron, magnesium, potassium, selenium, zinc), aloe vera juice, apple cider vinegar, coconut oil, CoQ10, cordyceps, echinacea, ginseng, grapefruit seed extract, graviola, spirulina; **Herbs:** boneset, chanca piedra, elder, eucalyptus, fenugreek, goldenseal, jaborandi, kudzu, lemongrass, licorice, macela, myrrh, olive leaf, pau d'arco, pleurisy root, sangre de grado, slippery elm, vervain, white oak, white willow, yohimbe

---

Insomnia – *(difficulty sleeping and/or falling asleep)*

Possible Factors – aging, antidepressants, asthma, alcohol, arthritis, anxiety, caffeine, calcium deficiency, cardiovascular disease, chocolate, depression, eating/working late, heartburn, hypoglycemia, hyperthyroidism, kidney disorders, medications, muscle aches, Parkinson's disease, restless leg syndrome, smoking, stress, sugar, traveling

Common Symptoms – daytime fatigue, irritability, lack of concentration, personality changes, trouble falling asleep, waking up at night or too early, weakened immune system, work productivity diminished

Helpful Nutrition – **Foods:** almonds, artichokes, asparagus, avocadoes, bananas, beets, berries, carrots, chicken, cucumber, dates, eggs, figs, grapefruit, grapes, leafy green vegetables, legumes, mangoes, melons, milk, nuts/seeds (raw), papayas, pineapples, sesame seeds, soy foods, sweet potatoes, tuna, turkey, turnips, watercress, whole grains, yogurt; **Spices:** cinnamon, cumin, dill, garlic, ginger, peppermint, turmeric; **Supplements:** (vitamins B-complex , C & D, calcium, choline, inositol, magnesium, manganese, potassium, zinc), graviola; **Herbs:** burdock, chamomile, goldenseal, hawthorn, lavender, motherwort, kava kava, oat straw, passionflower, skullcap, valerian

---

Irritable Bowl Syndrome (IBS) – *(digestive tract disorder marked by chronic abdominal pain)*

Possible Factors – acid/alkaline imbalance, alcohol, animal fats, antibiotics, antacids, butter, caffeine, chocolate, citrus fruits (acidic), coffee, colon cancer, dairy, diabetes, food allergies, gallbladder and pancreas disorders, laxatives, liver disorders, menstrual periods, metal toxicity, parasites, poor diet, seeds, smoking, soft drinks, stress, sugar

Common Symptoms – abdominal pain, anorexia, bloating, constipation, diarrhea, flatulence, mucus in stool, nausea

Helpful Nutrition – **Foods:** (*avoid raw vegetables/foods - only baked, boiled, broiled or steamed) apple sauce, artichokes, bananas, broccoli, carrots, cauliflower, figs, green tea (decaf), kelp, legumes, mangoes, olive oil, papayas, peaches, pineapples, pomegranate seeds, quinoa, squash, sweet potatoes, zucchini; **Spices:** cilantro, cinnamon, cumin, dill, fennel, garlic, ginger, mustard, oregano, parsley, peppermint, rosemary, turmeric; **Supplements:** (vitamins A, B-complex, calcium, magnesium, selenium, zinc), acidophilus, aloe vera juice, apple cider vinegar, bentonite, coconut oil, CoQ10, fish oil, flaxseed oil, grapefruit seed extract, milk thistle, psyllium, wheatgrass juice; **Herbs:** buchu, burdock, chamomile, goldenseal, horsetail, lemongrass, meadowsweet, passionflower, plantain, red clover, slippery elm, valerian, wild cherry, yerba buena, yerba mate

---

Jaundice – *(liver disorder characterized by the 'yellowing' of the eyes and skin)*

Possible Factors – cirrhosis, gallstones, hepatitis, obstructed bile flow, parasites, raw meat, tumors

Common Symptoms – fatigue, itching, nausea, rashes, vomiting, yellowing skin

Helpful Nutrition – **Foods:** alfalfa sprouts, almonds, apples, beets, bell peppers, berries, broccoli, brown rice, cabbage, carrots, eggs, leafy green vegetables, grapes (red), green tea (decaf), kale, lemons, limes, mangoes, melons, mushrooms, oat bran, onions, oranges, papayas, pineapples, pears, raisins, salmon, soy foods, spinach, sweet potatoes, tomatoes, whole grains; **Spices:** basil, cayenne pepper, cilantro, fennel, garlic, oregano, thyme, turmeric; **Supplements:** (vitamins A, B-complex, C & E, calcium, choline, magnesium), aloe vera juice, brewer's yeast, CoQ10, fish oil, flaxseed oil, grape seed extract, lecithin, milk thistle, St. John's wort, wheatgrass juice; **Herbs:** barberry, blessed thistle, boldo, boswellia, burdock, chamomile, chicory, dandelion, gentian, goldenseal, gotu kola, horsetail, Irish moss, licorice, Oregon grape, plantain, red clover, skullcap, vervain, wormwood, yellow dock

---

Kidney Disease (renal failure) – *(damage to the kidneys causing decreased function and/or kidney failure)*

Possible Factors – anemia, birth defects, chemotherapy, congestive heart failure, diabetes, environmental toxins, excessive protein, heavy metals, heredity, high blood pressure, liver disease, lupus, oxalate-rich foods (amaranth, beet greens, buckwheat, kale, okra, parsley, rhubarb, spinach, Swiss chard, watercress), poisonous mushrooms, venoms

Common Symptoms – abdominal/back/groin pain, acidosis, bone disorders, chills, bloody urine, difficulty/frequency urinating, edema, inflammation, kidney cysts, loss of appetite, nausea, nerve damage, vomiting

Helpful Nutrition – **Foods:** alfalfa sprouts, apples, asparagus, bananas, beans, bell peppers (red & yellow), berries, broccoli, cabbage, cauliflower, celery, cherries, cottage cheese (low-fat), cranberry juice, cucumber, distilled water w/ lemon, grapes (red), lemons, limes, millet, olive oil, onions, papayas, peaches, pomegranates, potatoes, pumpkin seeds, raisins, soy foods, watermelon, whole grains, yogurt (low-fat); **Spices:** cayenne pepper, garlic, parsley, turmeric; **Supplements:** (vitamins A, B-complex, C & E, calcium, magnesium, potassium, zinc), acidophilus, aloe vera juice, apple cider vinegar, coconut oil, cordyceps, fish oil, flaxseed oil, ginkgo biloba, milk thistle, wheatgrass juice; **Herbs:** barberry, buchu, butcher's broom, corn silk, dandelion, hydrangea, marshmallow, nettle, puncture vine, red clover, slippery elm, uva ursi

---

Kidney Stones – *(accumulation of crystallized mineral salts lodged in the urinary tract)*

Possible Factors – animal protein, dehydration, excessive calcium, heredity, lack of exercise, oxalate-rich foods (amaranth, beet greens, buckwheat, kale, okra, parsley, rhubarb, spinach, Swiss chard, watercress), poor diet, sugar, tomatoes, white flour

Common Symptoms – abdominal/back/groin pain, bloody urine, chills, difficulty/frequency urinating, sweating

Helpful Nutrition – **Foods:** alfalfa sprouts, apricots, avocados, brown rice, cantaloupe, carrots, cherries, cranberry juice (unsweetened), cucumber, distilled water w/ lemon, grapefruit, lemons, limes, onions, oranges, papayas, peaches, pomegranates, pumpkin, raisins, rye bread, soy foods, squash, water chestnuts, watermelon, wild rice; **Spices:** basil, cayenne pepper, dill, fennel, garlic, oregano, turmeric;

Supplements: (vitamins A, B-complex, C & E, magnesium, potassium, zinc), aloe vera juice, apple cider vinegar, coconut oil, cordyceps, fish oil, flaxseed oil, ginkgo biloba, grape seed extract, milk thistle, spirulina, wheatgrass juice; **Herbs:** barberry, buchu, chanca piedra, corn silk, dandelion, gotu kola, gravel root, hydrangea, marshmallow, nettle, puncture vine, white oak, uva ursi

---

Lactose Intolerance – *(inability of the lactase enzyme to absorb and digest lactose or milk sugar)*

Possible Factors – aging, heredity, injury to the small intestine

Common Symptoms – abdominal pain, bloating, celiac disease, cramps, colitis, diarrhea, flatulence, irritable bowel syndrome, nausea, vomiting, weight gain

Helpful Nutrition – **Foods:** apricots, barley, beans, beef, broccoli, broth, chicken, collard greens, dried fruits, figs, honey (raw), kale, leafy green vegetables, lentils, milk (almond, rice, soy, lactose-free), molasses, nuts/seeds (raw), oats (raw), olives, orange juice, pasta, peas, potatoes (plain), rhubarb, rice, salmon, sardines, soups, soy foods, spinach, yogurt; **Supplements:** (vitamins D & E, acidophilus, calcium, magnesium, zinc), acidophilus, fish oil, milk thistle

---

Leukemia – *(cancer of the blood, bone marrow, lymph system or spleen, characterized by the abnormal production of white blood cells)*

Possible Factors – Down's syndrome, environmental toxins, heredity, radiation exposure, virus

Common Symptoms – anemia, bleeding, bone and joint pain, bruising, difficulty breathing, enlarged liver or spleen, fatigue, fever, heavy perspiration, nosebleeds, paleness, slow-healing wounds, swollen lymph nodes, weight loss

Helpful Nutrition – **Foods:** alfalfa sprouts, bananas, beans, bell peppers (green & red), bok choy, broccoli, Brussels sprouts, cabbage, cauliflower, celery, collard greens, carrots, eggplant, humus, kale, leafy green vegetables, legumes, olive oil, onions, radishes, salmon, soy foods, spinach, squash, sweet potatoes, tomatoes, turnips, vegetables (steamed), watercress, whole grains; **Spices:** cayenne pepper, cinnamon, turmeric; **Supplements:** (vitamins A, B-complex, C & E, calcium, selenium), chlorophyll, fish oil, flaxseed oil, milk thistle, spirulina, St. John's wort; **Herbs:** calendula, dandelion, elder, horsetail, meadowsweet, nettle, wormwood

---

Lupus – *(inflammatory autoimmune disorder where the immune system develops antibodies that attack the body's own cells, tissues and organs)*

Possible Factors – alfalfa sprouts, birth control pills, environmental toxins, heredity, hormone imbalance, medications, pregnancy, stress, viral infection

Common Symptoms – abdominal pain, anemia, arthritis, bloody urine, difficulty breathing, fatigue, fever, hair loss, lesions, loss of appetite, mouth sores, muscle aches, nausea, poor circulation, rashes, Raynaud's disease, seizures, sensitivity to sunlight, swelling, ulcers, weight loss

Helpful Nutrition – **Foods:** apricots, asparagus, bananas, berries, broccoli, brown rice, Brussels sprouts, cabbage, canola oil, cantaloupe, carrots, cherries, eggs (free-range), herring, kale, kelp, kiwi, leafy green vegetables, mangosteen, molasses, oatmeal, olive oil, onions, pineapples, papayas, peaches, pomegranates, pumpkin, salmon, sardines, spinach, sweet potatoes, whole grains; **Spices:** garlic, ginger, turmeric; **Supplements:** (vitamins A, B-complex, C, D & E, calcium, magnesium, zinc), acidophilus, aloe vera juice, bromelain, coconut oil, CoQ10, fish oil, flaxseed oil, grape seed extract, milk thistle, royal jelly, wheatgrass juice; **Herbs:** burdock, feverfew, primrose, red clover

---

Macular Degeneration – *(progressive vision loss due to deterioration of the retina)*

Possible Factors – aging, atherosclerosis, environmental toxins, heredity, high blood pressure, sugar, white flour

Common Symptoms – arthritis, blurred/hazy vision, need for brighter lights, hallucinations, loss of vision

Helpful Nutrition – **Foods:** apricots, bananas, bell peppers (orange), berries, broccoli, cabbage, cantaloupe, carrot juice, cauliflower, collard greens, figs, grapefruit, green tea (decaf), kale, leafy green vegetables, mangoes, papayas, peaches, pineapples, prunes, pumpkin seeds, raisins, salmon, spinach, sunflower seeds, sweet potatoes, tomatoes, turnip greens, watercress, watermelon, zucchini; **Spices:** cayenne pepper; **Supplements:** (vitamins A, C & E, CoQ10, selenium, zinc), apple cider vinegar, fish oil, flaxseed oil, grape seed extract, wheatgrass juice; **Herbs:** bayberry, bilberry, eyebright, fenugreek

---

Measles (rubeola) – *(highly contagious paramyxovirus affecting the respiratory tract, eyes and skin)*

Possible Factors – airborne transmission, direct physical contact, droplet contact (sneezing, coughing)

Common Symptoms – bronchitis, cough, diarrhea, fever, inner ear infection, pneumonia, rashes, red bumps, runny nose, seizures, sore throat, strep throat, watery eyes

Helpful Nutrition – **Foods:** barley, berries, cantaloupe, cherries, herbal teas, grapes, kiwi, lemons, limes, mushrooms (shiitake), orange juice (diluted), papayas, pineapples, pomegranates, soups, strawberries, tomatoes, vegetable juices (organic); **Spices:** basil, cayenne pepper, garlic, ginger, oregano, parsley, turmeric; **Supplements:** (vitamins A, B-complex, C & E, calcium, magnesium, zinc), aloe vera juice, coconut oil, echinacea, grapefruit seed extract, spirulina; **Herbs:** chamomile, elder, goldenseal, licorice

---

Melanoma – *(most serious form of skin cancer that develops in the cells that produce melanin; the pigment that gives skin its color)*

Possible Factors – aging, environmental toxins, fair skin, heredity, radiation exposure, sunny or high-altitude climates, tanning beds

Common Symptoms – brown spots, bump on face/neck/ears, discolored mole, flat lesion, shiny bumps on body, skin discoloration

Helpful Nutrition – **Foods:** berries, broccoli, Brussels sprouts, cabbage, canola oil, cantaloupe, carrots, cauliflower, chives, green tea (decaf), honey (raw), kale, kelp, leafy green vegetables, lemons, limes, mackerel, mushrooms (maitake, reishi, shiitake), onions, peaches, pumpkin seeds, salmon, soy foods, spinach, squash, sweet potatoes, tomatoes, walnuts; **Spices:** basil, cayenne pepper, cilantro, ginger, mustard, oregano, parsley, rosemary, sage, thyme, turmeric; **Supplements:** (vitamins A, B-complex, C & E, calcium, choline, potassium, selenium, silicon, zinc), acidophilus, acidophilus, aloe vera juice, coconut oil, CoQ10, echinacea, fish oil, flaxseed oil, ginkgo biloba, ginseng, grape seed extract, milk thistle, wheatgrass juice; **Herbs:** astragalus, bilberry, burdock, cat's claw, comfrey (topically), dandelion, Irish moss, kudzu, marshmallow, nettle, oat straw, pau d'arco, red clover, rose, sarsaparilla, tea tree oil (topically)

Meningitis (viral) – *(viral infection in the blood affecting the brain, skull and spinal cord)*

Possible Factors – herpes, mosquito bites, mumps, viral infection

Common Symptoms – fatigue, fever, headache, rashes, sore throat, vomiting

Helpful Nutrition – **Foods:** barley, brown rice, cabbage, carrots, chicken (skinless), leafy green vegetables, mushrooms (maitake, reishi, shiitake), nuts/seeds (raw), olive oil, onions, pineapples, papayas, pumpkin seeds, salmon, turkey (skinless), walnuts, whole grains, yogurt; **Spices:** cayenne pepper, garlic; **Supplements:** (vitamins A & C, zinc), acidophilus, coconut oil, echinacea, fish oil, ginseng, St. John's wort; **Herbs:** astragalus, goldenseal, olive leaf

---

Menopause – *(end of the menstruation cycle and fertility for women)*

Possible Factors – aging, changes in estrogen and hormone levels

Common Symptoms – cardiovascular disease, emotional problems, fatigue, heart palpitations, hot flashes, insomnia, memory problems, night sweats, osteoporosis

Helpful Nutrition – **Foods:** alfalfa sprouts, amaranth, apples, asparagus, barley, beans, beets, bell peppers, broccoli, brown rice, cabbage, carrots, cauliflower, celery, cucumber, grapefruit, grapes (red), kelp, leafy green vegetables, molasses, nuts (raw), oat bran, olive oil, onions, oranges, pears, pineapples, plums, pomegranates, prunes, quinoa, raisins, raspberries, salmon, sardines, soy foods, strawberries, sweet potatoes, tomatoes, turkey, watercress, whole grains, yogurt; **Spices:** cayenne pepper, cilantro, cumin, dill, fennel, garlic, ginger, parsley, sage, turmeric; **Supplements:** (vitamins A, B-complex, C, D & E, boron, calcium, magnesium, potassium, selenium, zinc), CoQ10, fish oil, flaxseed oil, ginseng, lecithin, royal jelly, saw palmetto; **Herbs:** agnus castus, anise, black cohosh, blue cohosh, burdock, chaste tree, chickweed, cramp bark, damiana, dandelion, dong quai, goldenseal, gotu kola, kava kava, licorice, maca, macela, motherwort, muira puama, nettle, pleurisy root, primrose, puncture vine, red clover, sarsaparilla, valerian, vervain

---

Metal Toxicity – *(accumulation of heavy metals in the body: aluminum, arsenic, beryllium, cadmium, cobalt, copper, iron, lead, mercury, nickel, tin)*

Possible Factors – acid rain, aluminum cookware and foil, antacids, antiperspirants, auto exhaust, batteries, beer, birth control pills, bleached flour, candy, ceramics, childhood vaccines, cleaners, contact lens solution, cosmetics, dental fillings, diuretics, handling electrical parts, evaporated milk, fabric softeners, gasoline, hair dyes, industrial toxins, instant coffee, latex, medications, nasal sprays, paints, printer ink, processed meats, seafood, tap water, tattoos, tobacco, toothpaste (some), wood polishes

Common Symptoms – abdominal pain, Alzheimer's disease, anemia, constipation, decreased metabolism, diarrhea, difficulty concentrating, dizziness, dry skin, fatigue, hair loss, halitosis, headaches, insomnia, jaundice, joint pain, liver/brain/kidney damage, low blood pressure, lung cancer, memory loss, migraines, nausea, nervousness, neurological damage, paralysis, Parkinson's disease, peripheral vision loss, poisoning, rashes, respiratory problems, schizophrenia, spasms, thyroid dysfunction, vomiting, weakness

Helpful Nutrition – **Foods:** alfalfa sprouts, apples, artichokes, avocados, beans, beets, broccoli, cabbage, cantaloupe, cauliflower, celery, collard greens, cucumber, distilled water w/ lemon, fruit juices (organic), green tea (decaf), kale, kelp, leafy green vegetables, lemons, limes, mangoes, mangosteen, onions, radishes, soy foods, spinach, tomatoes, whole grains; **Spices:** cayenne pepper, fennel, garlic, ginger, parsley, turmeric; **Supplements:** (vitamins A, B-complex, C & E, calcium, selenium, sulfur, zinc), aloe vera juice, bentonite, brewer's yeast, chia seeds, coconut oil, flaxseed oil, psyllium, spirulina, wheatgrass juice; **Herbs:** burdock, chaparral, chicory, dandelion, goldenseal, lemongrass, oat straw

---

Migraine – *(neurological syndrome causing extremely painful, throbbing headaches)*

Possible Factors – alcohol (especially red wine), allergies, altitudes, aspirin, bright lights, caffeine, car exhaust, chemical imbalance, citrus fruits, dairy (cheese, milk, yogurt), eggs, excessive exercise, food allergies (chocolate, corn, peanuts, wheat, yeast), heredity, hormonal or nerve system changes, hypoglycemia, inactivity, insomnia or oversleeping, medications, MSG, nutritional deficiencies, poor circulation, processed meats, low serotonin levels, shellfish, sinus pressure, smoking, stress

Common Symptoms – coughing, debilitating pain, nausea, pain in temple, sensitivity to light/sound, severe headaches, slurred speech, vision problems, vomiting

Helpful Nutrition – **Foods:** almonds, almond milk, brown rice, cherries, halibut, leafy green vegetables, mackerel, mangosteen, olive oil, onions, peppermint tea, pineapples, quinoa, rice flour, puffed rice, salmon, sesame seeds, spinach, tuna, watercress; **Spices:** basil, cayenne pepper, cilantro, fennel, garlic, ginger, mustard, parsley, rosemary, thyme, turmeric; **Supplements:** (vitamins B-complex & C, calcium, magnesium), apple cider vinegar, bromelain, coconut oil, CoQ10, fish oil, flaxseed oil, ginkgo biloba, grape seed extract, milk thistle, royal jelly, saw palmetto, wheatgrass juice; **Herbs:** chamomile, fenugreek, feverfew, guarana, kudzu, lavender, lemongrass, passionflower, wood betony, wormwood, yerba buena, yucca

---

Mononucleosis (mono) – *(highly contagious Cytomegalovirus (CMV) or Epstein-Barr virus (EBV) affecting the respiratory system, lymphatic tissues and glands)*

Possible Factors – airborne transmission, direct physical contact, droplet contact (sneezing, coughing)

Common Symptoms – abdominal pain, depression, diarrhea, fatigue, fever, headaches, jaundice, loss of appetite, rashes, respiratory problems, sore throat, vomiting

Helpful Nutrition – **Foods:** alfalfa sprouts, avocadoes, barley, beans, berries, bran, broth, brown rice, cabbage, carrots, cherries, grapefruit, green tea (decaf), leafy green vegetables, mangoes, mushrooms (maitake, reishi, shiitake), oats (raw), olive oil, onions, papayas, pomegranates, salmon, soups, tofu, tomatoes, turkey, whole grains, yogurt; **Spices:** garlic, ginger, turmeric; **Supplements:** (vitamins A, B-complex, C, D & E, calcium, magnesium, potassium, zinc), acidophilus, coconut oil, echinacea, fish oil, flaxseed oil, grapefruit seed extract, milk thistle, spirulina, wheatgrass juice; **Herbs:** astragalus, cat's claw, dandelion, goldenseal, olive leaf, Oregon grape, pau d'arco

---

Multiple Sclerosis (MS) – *(inflammatory autoimmune disorder affecting the central nervous system)*

Possible Factors – environmental/industrial toxins, food allergies, gluten foods (barley, oats, rye, wheat), heredity, immune system malfunction, metal toxicity, poor diet, smoking, stress

Common Symptoms – anxiety, bladder/bowel problems, double/blurred vision, dizziness, fatigue, forgetfulness, loss of vision, muscle stiffness, numbness/weakness in the limbs, paralysis, sexual dysfunction, shock sensations w/ head movements, tremors

Helpful Nutrition – **Foods:** alfalfa sprouts, brown rice, cabbage, carrots, dill pickles, leafy green vegetables, lentils, mackerel, mangoes, nuts/seeds (raw), onions, papayas, salmon, soy foods, whole grains, zucchini; **Spices:** cayenne pepper, garlic, turmeric; **Supplements:** (vitamins A, B-complex, C, D, E & K, calcium, chromium, magnesium, manganese, phosphorous, potassium, selenium), acidophilus, brewer's yeast, chlorophyll, coconut oil, CoQ10, cordyceps, fish oil, flaxseed oil, grape seed extract, lecithin, milk thistle, St. John's wort, wheatgrass juice; **Herbs:** burdock, dandelion, goldenseal, pau d'arco, primrose, red clover, sarsaparilla, skullcap, valerian

---

Mumps – *(moderately contagious paramyxovirus that causes swelling of the salivary glands)*

Possible Factors – airborne transmission, direct physical contact, droplet contact (sneezing, coughing)

Common Symptoms – aching muscles, chills, fatigue, fever, headaches, loss of appetite, painful swallowing, sore throat, swollen saliva glands

Helpful Nutrition – **Foods:** asparagus, barley water, berries, broths, cantaloupe, grapes (red), herbal teas, kiwi, leafy green vegetables, mangoes, mushrooms (maitake, reishi, shiitake), oatmeal, orange juice (diluted), papayas, pineapples, pomegranates, vegetable juice, whole grains; **Spices:** basil, cayenne pepper, garlic, ginger, parsley, peppermint, turmeric; **Supplements:** (vitamins A, B-complex, C, & E, potassium, zinc), acidophilus, aloe vera juice, coconut oil, echinacea, grapefruit seed extract, peppermint oil (topically), spirulina; **Herbs:** chamomile, dandelion, elder, fenugreek, mullein, slippery elm

---

Muscle Cramps – *(painful, involuntary muscle contractions)*

Possible Factors – allergies, anemia, arteriosclerosis, arthritis, cholera, dehydration, electrolyte imbalance, excessive sitting or standing, heat exhaustion, high blood pressure, hormone imbalance, hypothyroidism, inactivity or overexertion, injury, medications, nutritional deficiencies, poor circulation, pregnancy, restless leg syndrome, smoking, varicose veins, vitamin E deficiency

Common Symptoms – headaches, muscle atrophy, severe muscle spasms or twitching

Helpful Nutrition – **Foods:** alfalfa sprouts, apple juice, apricots, asparagus, avocado, bananas, beans (lima), beets, bell peppers, berries, broccoli, cantaloupe, carrots, cherries, eggplant, halibut, honey (raw), kelp, kiwi, leafy green vegetables, lemons, limes, mangoes, mushrooms, olive oil, onions, oranges, peas, pineapples, pumpkin seeds, prunes, raisins, salmon, sesame seeds, spinach, squash, sunflower seeds, sweet potatoes, tomatoes, tuna, watermelon, zucchini; **Spices:** cayenne pepper, cilantro, garlic, ginger, peppermint, rosemary; **Supplements:** (vitamins A, B-complex, C, D & E, calcium, magnesium, potassium, zinc), apple cider vinegar, bromelain, coconut oil, CoQ10, fish oil, flaxseed oil, ginkgo biloba, grape seed extract, graviola, wheatgrass juice; **Herbs:** blessed thistle, blue cohosh, cramp bark, dong quai, elder, eucalyptus, horse chestnut, kava kava, meadowsweet, valerian, yerba buena

---

Narcolepsy – *(chronic neurological disorder characterized by excessive daytime sleepiness)*

Possible Factors – alcohol, brain infection/tumors, deficiency of certain brain chemicals, food allergies, heredity, metal toxicity, nutritional deficiencies, sugar, trauma

Common Symptoms – disruptive sleep patterns, excessive daytime sleepiness, fatigue, hallucinations, seizures, sleep paralysis

Helpful Nutrition – **Foods:** brown rice, cheese, chicken, eggs, fruits (organic), kelp, leafy green vegetables, legumes, muesli, nuts/seeds (raw), oats (raw), pasta, soy foods, wheat germ, whole grains; **Spices:** cayenne pepper, garlic, ginger; **Supplements:** (vitamins A, B-complex, C, D & E, calcium, choline, chromium, magnesium), brewer's yeast, CoQ10, fish oil, flaxseed oil, ginkgo biloba, lecithin, St. John's wort; **Herbs:** gotu kola

---

Nausea – *(discomfort or uneasy feeling in the stomach)*

Possible Factors – alcohol, anxiety, caffeine, food poisoning, junk food, medications, motion sickness, odors/fumes, over-eating, poor ventilation, smoking, stomach infection, stress

Common Symptoms – cold sweats, difficulty breathing, distress, dizziness, excessive saliva, fatigue, headaches, loss of appetite, queasiness, sleepiness, vomiting, weakness

Helpful Nutrition – **Foods:** almonds, apples, bananas, chicken broth, ginger ale, olives, whole grain crackers; **Spices:** basil, cinnamon, fennel, ginger, rosemary, peppermint; **Supplements:** (vitamins B-complex, magnesium), coconut oil, graviola, milk thistle; **Herbs:** anise, feverfew, meadowsweet

---

Obesity – *(accumulating excessive body fat)*

Possible Factors – constant hunger, depression, food allergies, food obsession, heredity, hypoglycemia, inactivity, overeating, poor diet, slow metabolism, stress, sugar, white flour

Common Symptoms – difficulty breathing, excessive weight, fatigue, medical complications

Helpful Nutrition – **Foods:** alfalfa sprouts, almonds, apples, avocados, bell peppers, berries (except cherries), broccoli, brown rice, cabbage, cantaloupe, carrot juice, cauliflower, celery, cucumber, figs, grapefruit, grapes (red), kelp, green tea (decaf), leafy green vegetables, lemons, limes, mangosteen, mushrooms (maitake, shiitake), oats (raw), olive oil, onions, peaches, prunes, radishes, salmon, soy foods, spinach, strawberries, watermelon, whole grains, yogurt (low-fat); **Spices:** cayenne pepper, cinnamon, fennel, garlic, ginger, mustard, parsley, turmeric; **Supplements:** (vitamins B-complex & C, boron, calcium, choline, inositol, magnesium, manganese, potassium, zinc), aloe vera juice, apple cider vinegar, chia seeds, coconut oil, CoQ10, cordyceps, fish oil, flaxseed oil, ginkgo biloba, grape seed extract, graviola, lecithin, milk thistle, psyllium, spirulina, wheatgrass juice; **Herbs:** boswellia, butcher's broom, corn silk, dandelion, gravel root, guarana, horsetail, hydrangea, hyssop, juniper, kudzu

Osteoporosis – *(degenerative disease where bone density is reduced and bones become brittle and weakened)*

Possible Factors – aging, alcohol, caffeine, calcium deficiency, carbonated drinks, chemotherapy, citrus fruits, excessive vitamin A, heredity, hormonal imbalance, inactivity, medications, smoking, sugar, yeast

Common Symptoms – back pain, brittle/easily-fractured bones, joint pain/swelling, loss of height, poor posture, weakened bones

Helpful Nutrition – **Foods:** alfalfa sprouts, almonds, amaranth, apples, apricots, asparagus, bananas, beans (baked, garbanzo & kidney), beets, broccoli, brown rice, Brussels sprouts, buckwheat, cashews, celery, cheese (cottage, ricotta, Swiss), chestnuts, collard greens, eggs, figs, hazelnuts, kale, kelp, leafy green vegetables, mackerel, mangosteen, milk (vitamin D fortified), mineral water w/ lemon, molasses, oats (raw), okra, olive oil, onions, orange juice (diluted), oysters, pasta, pineapples, pomegranates, prunes, pumpkin seeds, raisins, salmon, sardines, sesame seeds, soy foods, spinach, sunflower seeds, sweet potatoes, tomatoes, tomato juice, tuna, turnip greens, walnuts, wheat germ, whole grains, yogurt; **Spices:** cayenne pepper, dill, garlic, parsley, rosemary, sage, thyme, turmeric; **Supplements:** (vitamins A, B-complex, C, D, E & K, boron, calcium (chelated), copper, germanium, inositol, magnesium, manganese, molybdenum, potassium, silicon, sulfur, vanadium, zinc), apple cider vinegar, chia seeds, chondroitin, coconut oil, CoQ10, fish oil, flaxseed oil, glucosamine, royal jelly, wheatgrass juice; **Herbs:** black cohosh, boneset, chickweed, dandelion, feverfew, horsetail, nettle, oat straw, primrose, red clover, rose, yucca

---

Pancreatitis – *(accumulation of digestive enzymes causing inflammation of the pancreas impairing insulin production)*

Possible Factors – alcohol, bacterial infections, caffeine, cystic fibrosis, digestive disorders, eating large meals, gallstones, heredity, junk foods, medications, parasites, smoking, stress, sugar, white flour

Common Symptoms – abdominal pain, bloating, dehydration, fatty/oily stools, fever, flatulence, high blood pressure, jaundice, muscle aches, nausea, sweating, vomiting

Helpful Nutrition – **Foods:** almonds, bell peppers (red), blueberries, bran, brown rice, broccoli, Brussels sprouts, cabbage, canola oil, celery, cherries, chicken (skinless), eggplant, grapes (red), green tea (decaf), kale, kelp, leafy green vegetables, mangoes, mushrooms (reishi), olive oil, onions, papayas, pomegranates, pumpkin seeds, salmon, soy foods, spinach, tomatoes, turkey (skinless), walnuts, whole grains, yogurt (non-fat); **Spices:** basil, cayenne pepper, garlic, ginger, parsley, turmeric; **Supplements:** (vitamins A, B-complex, C & E, calcium, choline, chromium, inositol, magnesium, zinc), acidophilus, aloe vera juice, coconut oil, CoQ10, echinacea, fish oil, flaxseed oil, ginseng, goldenseal, grape seed extract, lecithin, milk thistle, royal jelly, wheatgrass juice; **Herbs:** burdock, dandelion, horsetail, mullein

---

Parasites (intestinal) – *(hard to detect parasitic invaders that live and feed off of the human body: hookworms, pinworms, roundworms, tapeworms, threadworms)*

Possible Factors – biting dirty fingernails, contact with infected children/pets, improper food handling, inhaling airborne parasite eggs, insect bites, poor sanitation, pork, raw fish, tap water, traveling, unclean lettuce/vegetables/fruits, undercooked meat, walking barefoot

Common Symptoms – abdominal pain, anal itching, bloating, bronchitis, chest pain, constipation, congestion, cough, diarrhea, fever, frequent colds/flu, heart burn, insomnia, loss of weight with continual hunger, low energy, muscle damage, rashes, restlessness, stomach pain or rumbling unrelated to hunger, vitamin B12 deficiency

Helpful Nutrition – **Foods:** beets, brown rice, carrots, cranberries, figs, grapefruit juice, leafy green vegetables, lemons, limes, onions, papayas, peaches, pineapples, pomegranate juice, pumpkin seeds, sesame seeds, sweet potato, squash, whole grains; **Spices:** basil, cayenne pepper, fennel, garlic, ginger, oregano, parsley, rosemary, sage, thyme, turmeric; **Supplements:** (vitamins B-complex & C, iron, zinc), acidophilus, aloe vera juice, apple cider vinegar, bentonite, bromelain, coconut oil, echinacea, flaxseed oil, grapefruit seed extract, graviola, psyllium; **Herbs:** agnus castus, birch, black cohosh, black walnut, cascara sagrada, chamomile, chaparral, clove, elder, goldenseal, licorice, mullein, olive leaf, pau d' arco, slippery elm, valerian, wood betony, wormwood, yellow dock

---

Parkinson's Disease – *(degenerative disorder affecting the central nervous system)*

Possible Factors – aging, alcohol, alkaloids, caffeine, environmental toxins (herbicides, pesticides, carbon monoxide), excessive carbs/dairy, head trauma, heredity, hot spices, excessive iron and manganese, male gender, processed foods, smoking, sugar, viral infections, vitamin D deficiency

Common Symptoms – constipation, drooling, hand tremors, loss of appetite, muscle/limb stiffness, nausea

Helpful Nutrition – **Foods:** almonds, bananas, beans (lima), bell peppers, bran, Brazil nuts, broccoli, brown rice, cabbage, carrot juice, green tea (decaf), kale, leafy green vegetables, legumes, mangoes, melons, mushrooms, mustard greens, onions, papayas, pasta, pecans, pumpkin seeds, prune juice, raisins, sesame seeds, spelt, spinach, tofu, walnuts, whole grains; **Spices:** cayenne pepper, garlic, ginger, sage, turmeric; **Supplements:** (vitamins A, B-complex, C, D & E, calcium, choline, magnesium, potassium, selenium), acidophilus, aloe vera juice, CoQ10, flaxseed oil, ginkgo biloba, ginseng, grape seed extract, milk thistle, royal jelly, wheatgrass juice; **Herbs:** burdock, dandelion, hyssop, licorice, mullein, passionflower, red clover, sarsaparilla

---

Pneumonia – *(inflammatory infection of the lungs)*

Possible Factors – alcohol, allergies, bacterial/fungal/parasitic/viral infections, diabetes, kidney failure, nutritional deficiencies, sickle cell disease, smoking, weakened immune system

Common Symptoms – abdominal pain, cardiovascular disease, chest pain, chills, cough, diarrhea, difficulty breathing, fatigue, fever, flu/cold, loss of appetite, measles, muscle aches, nausea, night sweats, phlegm, skin discoloration, sore throat, vomiting, weakness, wheezing

Helpful Nutrition – **Foods:** bell peppers, broccoli, broth, cabbage, carrot juice, cauliflower, celery, collard greens, fruit juices (organic), green tea (decaf), kale, leafy green vegetables, legumes, lemons, limes, melons, mushrooms (maitake, reishi, shiitake); **Spices:** cayenne pepper, garlic, ginger, turmeric; **Supplements:** (vitamins A, B-complex, C & E, zinc), acidophilus, aloe vera juice, apple cider vinegar, coconut oil, CoQ10, flaxseed oil, grape seed extract; **Herbs:** pleurisy root

---

Polyps – *(abnormal, potentially cancerous growths of skin tissue in the colon and rectum)*

Possible Factors – alcohol, caffeine, colitis, Crohn's disease, junk food, heredity, smoking

Common Symptoms – abdominal pain, allergies, constipation, diarrhea, poor diet, rectal bleeding

Helpful Nutrition – **Foods:** apples, apricots, bananas, barley, beets, bell peppers (red), berries, bran, broccoli, brown rice, Brussels sprouts, buckwheat, cabbage, cantaloupe, carrots, cauliflower, celery, cherries, figs, grapefruit, grapes, green tea (decaf), kale, kelp, leafy green vegetables, lemons, mangoes, mangosteen, millet, nectarines, nuts, oats (raw), olive oil, onions, papayas, peaches, pears, pineapples, plums, prunes, pumpkin seeds, quinoa, raisins, salmon, soy foods, spinach, squash, sweet potatoes, tomatoes, walnuts, watermelon, wheat germ, whole grains, yogurt, zucchini; **Spices:** basil, cayenne pepper, cilantro, cumin, fennel, garlic, mustard, oregano, parsley, rosemary, thyme, turmeric; **Supplements:** (vitamins A, B-complex, C, D & E, calcium, potassium, selenium, zinc), acidophilus, aloe vera juice, apple cider vinegar, CoQ10, cordyceps, echinacea, fish oil, flaxseed oil, grape seed extract, graviola, milk thistle, psyllium, wheatgrass juice; **Herbs:** jaborandi

---

Premenstrual Syndrome (PMS) – *(disorder affecting women's physical and emotional well being prior to menstruation)*

Possible Factors – food allergies, heredity, hormone imbalance, metabolism/physiological malfunction

Common Symptoms – abdominal pain/bloating, acne, anxiety, backache, cramps, depression, fatigue, headaches, hunger cravings, insomnia, irritability, joint pain, mood swings, water retention

Helpful Nutrition – **Foods:** apples, bananas, barley, beans, bell peppers, blackberries, bran, broccoli, Brussels sprouts, cabbage, cantaloupe, carrots, chicken, cranberry juice, eggs, green tea (decaf), halibut, kelp, leafy green vegetables, lemons, limes, mackerel, nuts/seeds, oatmeal, olive oil, onions, potatoes, prunes, quinoa, rice bran, salmon, soy foods, spinach, sweet potatoes, tuna, turkey, whole grains; **Spices:** cayenne pepper, dill, fennel, garlic, ginger, peppermint, turmeric; **Supplements:** (vitamins A, B-complex, C, D & E, calcium, choline, chromium, inositol, magnesium, manganese, zinc), acidophilus, fish oil, flaxseed oil, ginkgo biloba, ginseng, milk thistle, royal jelly, saw palmetto, spirulina; **Herbs:** calendula, chamomile, chaste tree, cramp bark, dong quai, kava kava, lady's mantle, licorice, macela, motherwort, muira puama, pleurisy root, primrose, squaw vine, valerian, vervain, white willow

---

Psoriasis – *(chronic autoimmune disorder affecting the skin and joints)*

Possible Factors – alcohol, heredity, low metabolism, medications, poison oak, stress, sunburn, surgery

Common Symptoms – arthritis, burning, itching, lesions, red patchy skin, scaly skin, swollen joints

Helpful Nutrition – **Foods:** apples, apricots, bananas, barley, bell peppers, berries, broccoli, brown rice, cabbage, canola oil, cantaloupe, carrots, cauliflower, celery, figs, kelp, oat bran, olive oil, onions, pomegranates, quinoa, salmon, soy foods, spinach, sweet potatoes, wheatgrass juice, whole grains; **Spices:** cayenne pepper, garlic, ginger, turmeric; **Supplements:** (vitamins A, B-complex, C, D & E, calcium, magnesium, selenium, zinc), aloe vera juice, apple cider vinegar, coconut oil, CoQ10, fish oil, flaxseed oil, lecithin, milk thistle, psyllium, wheatgrass juice; **Herbs:** borage, burdock, chickweed, comfrey (topically), dandelion, gotu kola, kudzu, lavender, marshmallow, nettle, Oregon grape, pau d'arco, primrose, red clover, sangre de grado, sarsaparilla, tea tree oil (topically), yellow dock

---

Raynaud's Disease – *(circulatory disorder making extremities hypersensitive to cold)*

Possible Factors – arteriosclerosis/atherosclerosis, arthritis, blood vessel spasms, carpal tunnel syndrome, cold temperatures, environmental/industrial toxins, injury, lack of exercise, lupus, medications, poor circulation, smoking, stress, surgery, thyroid disorders

Common Symptoms – gangrene, migraines, numbness, skin discoloration, skin ulcers

Helpful Nutrition – **Foods:** almonds, apples, avocados, berries, bran, broccoli, brown rice, Brussels sprouts, cabbage, cauliflower, green tea (decaf), leafy green vegetables, lemons, limes, olive oil, onions, oranges, plums, pomegranates, pumpkin seeds, salmon, watercress, watermelon, whole grains; **Spices:** cayenne pepper, fennel, garlic, ginger, rosemary, sage, turmeric; **Supplements:** (vitamins A, B-complex, C & E, calcium, germanium, magnesium, selenium, sulfur, zinc), aloe vera juice, coconut oil, CoQ10, fish oil, flaxseed oil, ginkgo biloba, ginseng, grape seed extract, milk thistle, royal jelly, wheatgrass juice; **Herbs:** black cohosh, blessed thistle, butcher's broom, gentian, gotu kola, hawthorn, hyssop, lemongrass, licorice, pau d'arco, primrose, skullcap, valerian, wintergreen, yohimbe

---

Rickets – *(vitamin D deficiency that leads to bone disease)*

Possible Factors – lack of sun exposure, pregnancy

Common Symptoms – anxiety, bowed legs, decreases calcium absorption, excessive sweating, muscle cramps, numbness of extremities, scoliosis, tooth decay, weakened bones

Helpful Nutrition – **Foods:** broccoli, clam chowder, cottage cheese, eggs (boiled), fruits/vegetables (raw), green tea, halibut, leafy green vegetables, liver, mackerel, mushrooms, nuts/seeds (raw), oats, potatoes, salmon, soy foods, spinach, whole grains, yogurt; **Spices:** garlic, turmeric; **Supplements:** (vitamins A, B-complex & D, boron, calcium, phosphorus, zinc), fish oil; **Herbs:** dandelion, nettle

---

Schizophrenia – *(mental disorder characterized by impaired sense of reality)*

Possible Factors – alcohol, caffeine, excessive fats, heredity, nutritional deficiencies, stress, sugar

Common Symptoms – confusion, delusions, depression, difficulty speaking, fatigue, hallucinations, lack of interest, loss of memory, low emotional output, mood swings, suicide, violent outbursts

Helpful Nutrition – **Foods:** beets, bran, broccoli, carrots, corn, chicken (breast), eggs, halibut, kelp, leafy green vegetables, potatoes, salmon, soy foods, sweet potatoes, sunflower seeds, tomatoes, tuna, turkey, whole grains; **Spices:** cayenne pepper, cinnamon, garlic, ginger, turmeric; **Supplements:** (vitamins B-complex, C & E, calcium, magnesium, manganese, zinc), aloe vera juice, brewer's yeast, fish oil, flaxseed oil, ginkgo biloba, ginseng, grape seed extract, wheatgrass juice; **Herbs:** passionflower

---

Scurvy – *(vitamin C deficiency that compromises collagen formation)*

Possible Factors – vitamin C deficiency

Common Symptoms – anemia, bleeding gums, bruising, fatigue, joint pain and/or swelling, loss of hair/teeth, muscle weakness, slow-healing wounds, spotty skin, weakened collagen in tissues/bones

Helpful Nutrition – **Foods:** alfalfa sprouts, artichokes, asparagus, avocados, bananas, bell peppers, berries, broccoli, Brussels sprouts, cabbage, cantaloupe, carrots, cauliflower, cherries, corn, cucumber, grapefruit, grapes, green tea, kale, kiwi, leafy green vegetables, lemons, limes, mangoes, mangosteen, melons, olive oil, onions, orange juice, papayas, peaches, pears, peas, pineapples, pomegranates, radishes, spinach, strawberries, sweet potatoes, tangerines, tomatoes, watercress, watermelon, yogurt, zucchini; **Spices:** cayenne pepper, fennel, parsley, peppermint; **Supplements:** (vitamin C), apple cider vinegar, coconut oil, fish oil, grape seed extract, graviola, wheatgrass juice; **Herbs:** burdock, dandelion, eyebright, fenugreek, mullein, nettle, plantain, red clover

---

Senility – *(a form of dementia that is marked by a progressive decline in brain function)*

Possible Factors – aging, AIDS, alcohol, atherosclerosis, diabetes, hypothyroidism, liver/kidney failure, metal toxicity, multiple sclerosis, nutritional deficiencies, stress, stroke

Common Symptoms – agitation, depression, cognitive decline, difficulty speaking and/or thinking, fear of being alone, frustration, hallucinations, malnutrition, memory loss, mood swings, paranoia

Helpful Nutrition – **Foods:** apples, beets, bran, broccoli, brown rice, buckwheat, carrots, grapes (red), green tea (decaf), kale, kelp, leafy green vegetables, mushrooms (maitake, reishi, shiitake), nuts/seeds (raw), oat bran, olive oil, pomegranates, rice bran, salmon, spinach, Swiss cheese, tuna, whole grains, yogurt (low-fat); **Spices:** cayenne pepper, cinnamon, cumin, fennel, garlic, ginger, rosemary, sage, thyme, turmeric; **Supplements:** (vitamins B-complex, C & E, CoQ10, boron, choline, inositol, iodine, phosphorus, silicon, zinc), aloe vera juice, apple cider vinegar, bentonite, chia seeds, fish oil, flaxseed oil, ginkgo biloba, ginseng, grape seed extract, lecithin, royal jelly, wheatgrass juice; **Herbs:** blessed thistle, blue cohosh, eyebright, gotu kola, guarana, hyssop, primrose

---

Sexually Transmitted Diseases (STD's) – *(disease passed through sexual contact – Chlamydia, crabs, genital herpes, gonorrhea, hepatitis, HIV, HPV, syphilis)*

Possible Factors – bacterial/parasitic/viral infection, sharing clothes/beds, unprotected sex

Common Symptoms – abdominal pain, blisters, body aches, fatigue, fever, genital warts, night sweats, painful urination, scaly rashes, sexual pain, skin discoloration, swollen glands

Helpful Nutrition – **Foods:** alfalfa sprouts, green tea, kelp, leafy green vegetables; **Spices:** garlic, turmeric; **Supplements:** (vitamins B-complex, C, E & K, zinc), acidophilus, aloe vera juice, coconut oil, CoQ10, echinacea, flaxseed oil, grape seed extract, grapefruit seed extract, wheatgrass juice; **Herbs:** astragalus, cedar, chanca piedra, chickweed, goldenseal, pau d'arco, red clover, yucca

---

Shingles (herpes zoster) – *(reactivation of the highly contagious chickenpox virus (Varicella-zoster) that causes painful skin rashes)*

Possible Factors – chemotherapy, chickenpox, spinal cord injury, stress, weakened immune system

Common Symptoms – abdominal pain, blindness, blisters, burning sensation, chills, fever, headache, itching, kidney/liver/lung disorders, loss of hearing, pain, paralysis, rashes

Helpful Nutrition – **Foods:** alfalfa sprouts, bananas, brown rice, grapefruit, green tea (decaf), kelp, leafy green vegetables, pomegranates, sweet potatoes, whole grains; **Spices:** cayenne pepper, garlic, turmeric; **Supplements:** (vitamins A, B-complex, C, D & E, calcium, magnesium, zinc), acidophilus, brewer's yeast, chlorophyll, coconut oil, CoQ10, echinacea, flaxseed oil, grape seed extract, grapefruit seed extract, milk thistle, St. John's wort, wheatgrass juice; **Herbs:** astragalus, burdock, chamomile, dandelion, goldenseal, licorice, oat straw, olive leaf, red clover, rose, valerian

Sinusitis – *(inflammation of the nasal cavity and sinus passages)*

Possible Factors – air pollution, allergies, bacterial/fungal/viral infection, dairy, face trauma, mold, smoking, stress, sugar, toxic fumes, weakened immune system

Common Symptoms – bad breath, cough, decreased sense of smell, difficulty breathing, ear pain, facial/nasal pain, fatigue, headache, insomnia, nausea, snoring, sore throat, tooth pain

Helpful Nutrition – **Foods:** broccoli, cabbage, cauliflower, fruit/vegetable juices (organic), grapefruit, herbal teas, horseradish, kelp, mushrooms (maitake), oats (raw), olive oil, onions, soups, whole grains; **Spices:** cayenne pepper, garlic, ginger, parsley, turmeric; **Supplements:** (vitamins A, B-complex, C & E, zinc), acidophilus, apple cider vinegar, bromelain, CoQ10, flaxseed oil, grape seed extract, wheatgrass juice; **Herbs:** anise, bayberry, cat's claw, fenugreek, marshmallow, mullein, nettle, olive leaf, red clover, rose

---

Stress – *(caused by changes in mental, physical and social aspects of life)*

Possible Factors – alcohol, anxiety, birth of a child, crowds, death of family member/friend, holidays, illness, injury, lack of sleep, money/relationship problems, moving, new job, smoking, surgery, traffic, work deadlines

Common Symptoms – cold hands, decreased sexual drive, difficulty breathing, fatigue, headaches, high blood pressure, insomnia, loss of appetite, memory loss, nausea, social withdrawal, teeth grinding

Helpful Nutrition – **Foods:** avocados, baked potatoes, bananas, berries, broccoli, brown rice, cabbage, carrots, cauliflower, chicken, corn, fruit juices (organic), leafy green vegetables, mushrooms (maitake, reishi, shiitake), oat bran, onions, salmon, whole grains, yogurt; **Spices:** cayenne pepper, garlic, ginger, peppermint; **Supplements:** (vitamins B-complex, C & E, calcium, inositol, magnesium, potassium, selenium, zinc), aloe vera juice, brewer's yeast, coconut oil, CoQ10, fish oil, flaxseed oil, ginkgo biloba, ginseng, grape seed extract, lecithin, milk thistle, psyllium, royal jelly, St. John's wort, wheatgrass juice; **Herbs:** ashwagandha, bilberry, boneset, chamomile, chaste tree, dong quai, hawthorn, hops, kava kava, lavender, lemongrass, motherwort, passionflower, skullcap, valerian

---

Tendinitis – *(inflammation of the tendons - shoulders, wrists, elbows, heels and groin)*

Possible Factors – aging, arthritis, excessive activities causing wear and tear, physical strain

Common Symptoms – inflammation, limited motion, pain, redness, swelling

Helpful Nutrition – **Foods:** alfalfa sprouts, artichokes, asparagus, avocados, beets, bell pepper, broccoli, brown rice, cherries, eggs, green tea, kale, kelp, oats, olive oil, onions, papayas, pineapples, pomegranates, pumpkin seeds, salmon, soy foods, spinach, sweet potatoes, tomatoes, walnuts, watermelon, whole grains; **Spices:** basil, cayenne pepper, cilantro, cinnamon, garlic, ginger, oregano, parsley, peppermint, rosemary, turmeric; **Supplements:** (vitamins A, B-complex, C & E, calcium, magnesium, selenium, zinc), acidophilus, aloe vera juice, apple cider vinegar, bromelain, chondroitin, coconut oil, copper, CoQ10, fish oil, flaxseed oil, ginkgo biloba, glucosamine, grape seed extract, saw palmetto, St. John's wort, wheatgrass juice; **Herbs:** burdock, dandelion, fenugreek, horsetail, primrose

---

Tooth Decay – *(gradual erosion of teeth from bacteria in plaque)*

Possible Factors – acidic saliva, bacteria, frequent snacking, junk foods, lack of oral hygiene, sugar

Common Symptoms – teeth sensitive to cold, heat and consuming sugars

Helpful Nutrition – **Foods:** cranberry juice (unsweetened), fruits/vegetables (raw), green tea, pomegranates, raisins; **Spices:** mustard, peppermint, thyme, turmeric; **Supplements:** (vitamins A, B-complex, C, D, E & K, calcium, magnesium, zinc), acidophilus, aloe vera juice, apple cider vinegar, coconut oil, CoQ10, grape seed extract, St. John's wort, wheatgrass juice, **Herbs:** bay leaf, chaparral, licorice, myrrh

---

Tuberculosis – *(highly contagious, airborne bacterial disease primarily of the lungs)*

Possible Factors – bacteria inhalation, crowded conditions, poor ventilation, weakened immune system

Common Symptoms – bloody phlegm, bone/intestinal/kidney/liver dysfunction, chest pain, cough, difficulty breathing, fatigue, fever, insomnia, loss of appetite, night sweats, weight loss

Helpful Nutrition – **Foods:** alfalfa sprouts, asparagus, carrot juice, kefir, kelp, leafy green vegetables, nuts/seeds (raw), pineapple juice, pomegranates, potato juice (raw), salmon, sweet potatoes, yogurt (sugar free), whole grains; **Spices:** cayenne pepper, garlic, peppermint, sage, thyme, turmeric; **Supplements:** (vitamins A, B-complex, C, D & E, calcium, magnesium, selenium, zinc), acidophilus, aloe vera juice, coconut oil, CoQ10, echinacea, flaxseed oil, grape seed extract, wheatgrass juice; **Herbs:** butcher's broom, calendula, chamomile, goldenseal, licorice, marshmallow, mullein, pau d'arco, plantain

---

Tumor – *(abnormal growth of body tissue either benign (non-cancerous) or malignant (cancerous) that forms a solid lesion)*

Possible Factors – alcohol, animal protein, environmental toxins, heredity, lack of exercise, obesity, poor diet, radiation, smoking, stress, sugar, sun exposure, white flour

Common Symptoms – constipation, coughing, fatigue, fever, loss of appetite, sweating, weight loss

Helpful Nutrition – **Foods:** almonds, apples, apricots, beets, berries, broccoli, brown rice, cabbage, carrots, cashews, cauliflower, celery, grapefruit, honey (raw), kelp, leafy green vegetables, mangoes, mangosteen, mushrooms (shiitake), nuts/seeds (raw), onions, peaches, pineapples, salmon, soy foods, sweet potatoes, tomatoes, whole grains, yogurt; **Spices:** cayenne pepper, cumin, garlic, mustard, parsley, peppermint, sage, thyme, turmeric; **Supplements:** (vitamins A, B-complex, C & E, zinc), aloe vera juice, apple cider vinegar, coconut oil, CoQ10, cordyceps, fish oil, flaxseed oil, grape seed extract, ginseng, graviola, milk thistle, psyllium, royal jelly, wheatgrass juice; **Herbs:** barberry, burdock, cat's claw, chuchuhuasi, dandelion, pau d'arco, red clover, sangre de grado, yellow dock

---

Ulcer (peptic) – *(open sores that form on the inside lining of the stomach, esophagus or small intestine)*

Possible Factors – acid reflux, alcohol, aspirin, bacterial infections, caffeine, chocolate, coffee, excessive sodium, fried foods, ibuprofen, naproxen, smoking, spices, stress, sugar, white flour

Common Symptoms – blood in vomit or bowel movements, chest pain, constipation, fatigue, frequent belching or hiccupping, heartburn, indigestion, loss of appetite, nausea, vomiting, weight loss

Helpful Nutrition – **Foods:** alfalfa sprouts, apples, apricots, artichokes, avocado, bananas, barley, beets, berries, broccoli (steamed), brown rice, cabbage, carrots (steamed), cantaloupe, celery, cranberry juice, cottage cheese, dates, eggs, honey (raw), kelp, leafy green vegetables, mangoes, mangosteen, melons, millet, olive oil, onions, papayas, pears, peas, pineapples, plums, potatoes, salmon, soy foods, squash, sweet potatoes, yogurt; **Spices:** cayenne pepper, garlic, peppermint, sage, turmeric; **Supplements:** (vitamins A, B-complex, C, E & K, iron, zinc), acidophilus, aloe vera juice, apple cider vinegar, bentonite, bromelain, coconut oil, CoQ10, fish oil, flaxseed oil, grape seed extract, ginseng, graviola, psyllium, royal jelly, St. John's wort, wheatgrass juice; **Herbs:** astragalus, bayberry, cat's claw, fenugreek, goldenseal, hops, Irish moss, kava kava, meadowsweet, pau d'arco, slippery elm

---

Urinary Tract Infection – *(bacterial infection of the intestine causing inflammation of the bladder)*

Possible Factors – acidic foods (citrus fruits, tomatoes), alcohol, caffeine, chocolates, diabetes, diaphragm usage, obstruction of urinary tract, pregnancy, sexual intercourse, spices

Common Symptoms – abdominal and/or lower back pain, bloody urine, burning sensation, fever, frequent urination, nausea, urine odor, vomiting

Helpful Nutrition – **Foods:** beets, blueberries, broccoli, cauliflower, celery, cranberry juice (unsweetened), distilled water w/ lemon, salmon, watermelon, yogurt; **Spices:** cayenne pepper, garlic, ginger, oregano, parsley, thyme, turmeric; **Supplements:** (vitamins A, B-complex, C, D & E, calcium, magnesium, potassium, zinc), acidophilus, brewer's yeast, coconut oil, fish oil, saw palmetto, St. John's wort, wheatgrass juice; **Herbs:** astragalus, bilberry, birch, buchu, burdock, butcher's broom, cedar, chamomile, chanca piedra, chicory, corn silk, dandelion, goldenseal, gotu kola, gravel root, hydrangea, Irish moss, jatoba, juniper, kava kava, marshmallow, mullein, nettle, Oregon grape, plantain, puncture vine, pygeum, red clover, rose, saw palmetto, slippery elm, uva ursi

---

Vaginitis (yeast infection) – (*bacterial or fungal infection causing inflammation of the vaginal lining and mucous membranes*)

Possible Factors – acidic foods (citrus fruits, tomatoes), antibiotics, birth control pills, deodorants, diabetes, excessive douching, gluten foods (barley, oats, rye, wheat), hormonal changes, medications, menopause, poor hygiene, pregnancy, STD's, sugar, tight clothing, vitamin B deficiency

Common Symptoms – itching, painful sexual intercourse, painful urination, vaginal discharge/bleeding

Helpful Nutrition – **Foods:** brown rice, buckwheat, chicken (skinless), grapefruit, millet, salmon, vegetables (raw or steamed), yogurt; **Spices:** cayenne pepper, cinnamon, garlic, oregano, sage, turmeric; **Supplements:** (vitamins A, B-complex, C, D, E & K, calcium, magnesium, selenium, zinc), acidophilus, aloe vera gel (topically), aloe vera juice, apple cider vinegar (topically), coconut oil, CoQ10, echinacea, fish oil, flaxseed oil, grapefruit seed extract, wheatgrass juice; **Herbs:** barberry, chamomile, dandelion, jatoba, olive leaf, pau d'arco, sangre de grado, tea tree oil

---

Varicose Veins – *(enlarged, lumpy, bluish looking veins primarily on the legs and feet)*

Possible Factors – blood valve malfunction, heavy lifting, lack of exercise, long periods of sitting or standing, obesity, poor circulation

Common Symptoms – aching/throbbing legs, bluish veins, heaviness sensation, hemorrhoids, itching, leg sores, muscle cramps, skin ulcers, swelling

Helpful Nutrition – **Foods:** blackberries, bran, cherries, fruit juices (organic), mackerel, oats (raw), onions, pineapples, vegetables, salmon, tuna, whole grains; **Spices:** cayenne pepper, garlic, ginger, rosemary, turmeric; **Supplements:** (vitamins A, B-complex, C, D E & K, calcium, magnesium, zinc), aloe vera gel (topically), aloe vera juice, brewer's yeast, bromelain, CoQ10, fish oil, flaxseed oil, ginkgo biloba, grape seed extract, psyllium, wheatgrass juice; **Herbs:** bayberry, butcher's broom, gotu kola, horse chestnut, lemongrass, oat straw, white oak

---

Warts – *(highly contagious human papillomavirus (HPV) causing small tumorous growths)*

Possible Factors – contact with infected person, heredity

Common Symptoms – clusters of bumps, raised/scaly bumps, red bumps

Helpful Nutrition – **Foods:** asparagus, avocado, bananas, broccoli, citrus fruits, eggs, grapefruit, legumes, lemons, limes, mushrooms (reishi, shiitake), nuts/seeds, oats, onions, pomegranates, spinach, Swiss chard, tomatoes, watermelon; **Spices:** garlic, ginger, parsley, peppermint, turmeric; **Supplements:** (vitamins A, B-complex, C & E, zinc), aloe vera juice, coconut oil, grapefruit seed extract, wheatgrass juice; **Herbs:** astragalus, black walnut, chickweed, lemongrass, tea tree, wintergreen

---

Weakened Immune System – *(immune system malfunction increasing susceptibility to health disorders)*

Possible Factors – aging, alcohol, antibiotics, autoimmune disorders, bacterial/viral infections, blood transfusions (HIV/AIDS), cancer, chemotherapy, dehydration, drugs, heredity, influenza, lack of exercise, lack of sleep, nutritional deficiencies, smoking, stress

Common Symptoms – allergies, coughing, diarrhea, fatigue, fever, headaches, nausea, pneumonia, respiratory problems, skin lesions, swollen lymph nodes, sweating, weight loss

Helpful Nutrition – **Foods:** apples, asparagus, bananas, beans, beets, berries, broccoli, brown rice, Brussels sprouts, cabbage, cantaloupe, carrot juice, cauliflower, grapefruit, green tea (decaf), honey (raw), kale, kelp, leafy green vegetables, lemons, limes, melons, mushrooms (maitake, reishi, shiitake), nuts/seeds (raw), olive oil, onions, oranges, papayas, peaches, pineapples, pomegranates, pumpkin seeds, salmon, soy foods, spinach, sweet potatoes, turkey, tomatoes (cooked), watermelon, whole grains, yogurt; **Spices:** cayenne pepper, cumin, fennel, garlic, ginger, mustard, oregano, parsley, rosemary, turmeric; **Supplements:** (vitamins A, B-complex, C, D & E, chromium, germanium, manganese, selenium, silicon, sulfur, zinc), aloe vera juice, apple cider vinegar, bentonite, coconut oil, CoQ10, cordyceps, echinacea, fish oil, flaxseed oil, ginkgo biloba, ginseng, milk thistle, royal jelly, spirulina, St. John's wort, wheatgrass juice; **Herbs:** ashwagandha, astragalus, bayberry, burdock, cat's claw, eyebright, licorice, macela, myrrh, pau d'arco, puncture vine, red clover, yerba mate

---

Wrinkles – *(skin losing its elasticity usually as a result of aging)*

Possible Factors – aging, alcohol, caffeine, environmental toxins, facial expressions, fair skin, heredity, lack of exercise, poor nutrition, smoking, stress, sun exposure, tanning booths

Common Symptoms – crows feet around eyes, dry/thinning skin, wisdom

Helpful Nutrition – **Foods:** alfalfa sprouts, almonds, apples, beans, berries, bran, brown rice, cranberry juice, cucumber, leafy green vegetables, millet, olive oil, onions, pomegranates, pumpkin seeds, salmon, whole grains; **Spices:** garlic, ginger, parsley, thyme, turmeric; **Supplements:** (vitamins A, B-complex, C, D & E, calcium, magnesium, zinc), aloe vera gel (topically), aloe vera juice, coconut oil, CoQ10, fish oil, flaxseed oil, grape seed extract, wheatgrass juice; **Herbs:** acerola, borage, burdock root, chamomile, comfrey, lemongrass, oat straw, witch hazel

Part Five

Appendix

~ Glossary ~

A

Absorption – the process of assimilating nutrients into the body

Acetic Acid – the active ingredient in vinegar

Acid – compounds that have a low pH, are corrosive and sour to the taste

Acidophilus – a probiotic containing friendly bacteria that helps maintain digestive health

Acidosis – excessive acidity in the body

Adaptogen – herbal substances that reduce stress and produce beneficial adjustments in the body

Adrenal gland – a pair of glands responsible for regulating stress response

Allergen – a substance that creates an allergic reaction

Allergy – the immune systems negative response to foreign substance in the body

Allyl sulfides – phytonutrients that help detoxify the body

Alpha-carotene – a phytonutrient found in carrots that is beneficial for eye health

Alpha-linolenic acid (ALA) – omega-3 essential fatty acid found in flaxseed, pumpkin & soybean oils

Amino acid – nitrogen and carbon-based organic compounds that build protein and muscle

Amylases – enzymes that need calcium to break down carbohydrates into glucose

Anabolic – substance that helps convert nutrition into building and repairing muscle tissues in the body

Antacid – a substance that neutralizes stomach acid

Antibiotic – chemotherapeutic substance that inhibits the growth of bacteria, fungus or parasites

Antibody – immune system protein that combats bacteria, fungus and other foreign substances

Antigen – a substance that provokes the creation of antibodies

Antihistamine – a substance that binds with histamine receptors and reduces the effects of histamines

Antioxidant – a substance that minimizes free radical damage to the heart, arteries, and tissues, such as vitamins, minerals and nutrients

Arachidonic acid (AA) – an omega-6 essential fatty acid found in eggs, meat, poultry and shellfish

Ascorbic acid – the organic compound known as vitamin C

Autoimmune disorder – condition where the immune system reacts negatively to the body (Addison's disease, arthritis, Celiac disease, colitis, Crohn's disease, Cushing's syndrome, Type 1 diabetes, dermatitis, fibromyalgia, hepatitis, hyperthyroidism (Graves' disease), irritable bowel syndrome (IBS), lupus, multiple sclerosis (MS), pancreatitis, Parkinson's disease, psoriasis, Raynaud's phenomenon)

B

Bacteria – microorganisms that can be both beneficial and detrimental to human health

Beta carotene – phytonutrient with antioxidant properties the body uses to produce vitamin A, found in broccoli, carrots, collard greens, kale, pumpkin, spinach and sweet potatoes

Bio-availability – the ease of which nutrients can be absorbed into the body

Bioflavonoid – a group of active substances essential for the absorption of vitamin C

Blood clots – a natural process where blood cells for a clump to stop bleeding

Blood sugar – concentration of glucose in the blood

C

Capillaries – blood vessels that manage the exchange of nutrients and waste in the bloodstream

Carbohydrate – organic substances that are the main source of energy in our diet

Carcinogen – a toxic substance capable of producing cancer

Carotene – a substance that is converted into vitamin A in the body

Cartenoids – phytonutrients that have antioxidant properties

Cellulose – an organic carbohydrate from fruits and vegetables

Chelation – chemical process where molecules bind to a mineral atom increasing its bio-availability

Chelation therapy – the introduction of substances into the body to remove heavy metals

Chlorophyll – the green pigment in plants that is vital for photosynthesis; converting light into energy

Cholesterol – steroid metabolite compound including lipids (fats) naturally produced by the body, a structural component of cell membranes, helps absorption of fatty acids; HDL (good) and LDL (bad)

Chondroitin – derivative of glucosamine that strengthens connective tissues and protects against arthritis

Chronic illness – a disorder or condition that is persistent and long lasting

Citric acid – organic acid found in citrus fruits

Coconut oil – natural oil from coconuts, nature's best source of lauric acid, helps eliminate parasites, yeast infections, viruses, skin disorders and enhances the immune system

Coenzyme – a substance that works with enzymes to promote normal enzyme activity

Colic – abdominal pain caused by spasms or obstructions in the intestines or bile ducts

Complete protein – a protein that contains all 8 essential amino acids

Complex carbohydrate – a carbohydrate that provides fiber and slowly releases sugar into the body

Congenital – a condition present at birth, but not always inherited

Conjugated Linoleic Acid (CLA) – a naturally occurring fatty-acid that helps reduce body fat

Coronary Artery Disease (CAD) – narrowing of the small blood vessels that supply blood and oxygen to the heart (arteriosclerosis, atherosclerosis)

Cortisol – one of the main catabolic hormones in the body

Creatine – a high-energy compound in muscle cells which stores energy and increases strength

Cruciferous – 'cross-shaped' blossoms that help prevent colon cancer (broccoli, cabbage, cauliflower)

D

Dementia – a progressive decline in mental function and health, either temporary or permanent

Detoxification – process of eliminating toxic substances from the body

Dithiolthiones – phytonutrients in vegetables that increase enzyme levels and reduce the risk of cancer

Diuretic – substance that increases urine flow

Docosahexaenoic acid (DHA) – an omega-3 essential fatty acid found in marine micro-algae, anchovies, cod, mackerel, salmon and tuna

E

EDTA (ethylenediaminetetraacetic acid) – amino acid used in chelation therapy

Eicosapentaenoic acid (EPA) – an omega-3 essential fatty acid found in cod, salmon, sardines and tuna

Elastin – proteins that support tissue elasticity

Electrolytes (potassium, sodium and chloride) – soluble substances containing free ions that are capable of conducting electric impulses throughout the body

Ellagic acid – a phytonutrient that helps eliminate free radicals from the body

Endorphin – a hormone-like compound in the brain that binds to opiate receptors and reduces pain

Enzyme – a protein catalyst that manages or increases chemical reactions in the body

Essential Fatty Acids (EFA's) – amino acids that cannot be synthesized by the body and must be supplied by foods or supplements

F

Fat-soluble – the ability to dissolve in fats and oils

Fatty acid – a carboxylic acid derived from natural fats and oils

Fiber – indigestible plant matter that helps eliminate toxins from the body (fruits, vegetables, nuts, legumes, whole grains)

Flatulence – accumulation of gas in the digestive tract and stomach

Flavonoid – a class of metabolite substances found in plants that help protect against cancer

Free radicals – highly reactive molecules produced during the metabolism of food and energy that contribute to aging, cell damage or disease

Fructose – **a s**ugar found in fruit that has a low glycemic index

Fungus (mold, mushrooms, yeast) – a class of organisms capable of causing severe disease

G

Gamma-linolenic acid (GLA) – an omega-6 essential fatty acid found in borage & primrose oil

Gastritis – inflammation of the stomach lining

Gastroenteritis – inflammation of the mucus lining in the gastrointestinal tract

Gastrointestinal disorders – disorders of the esophagus, stomach, intestines, liver, colon, gallbladder and pancreas (colitis, colon polyps, constipation, diverticulitis, hemorrhoids, irritable bowel syndrome)

Genetics – the biological science of heredity

Gastroesophageal Reflux Disease (GERD) – term for acid reflux or heartburn

Gland – an organ that synthesizes substances for release into the bloodstream

Glucose – a simple sugar in the blood that is the major energy source for the body's cells and functions

Glucosamine – an amino sugar that helps protect against arthritis and osteoporosis, repairs cartilage and strengthens tendons, usually combined in supplement form with chondroitin

Gluten – a protein found in oats, wheat, barley and rye

Glycemic Index (GI) – measure of how much food raises blood sugar levels as compared to white bread, which has a GI of 100 (the lower the number the less insulin is released by the body)

Glycerol – a three-carbon sugar of which fatty acids attach to form triglycerides

Glycogen – the main form of glucose stored in the body, then converts back to glucose to supply energy

Growth Hormone (GH) – a hormone that is released by the pituitary gland that promotes muscle growth and the breakdown of body fat for energy, subsides with age

H

HDL cholesterol (high-density lipoprotein) – known as *good cholesterol,* it helps clear fat from the bloodstream and indicates a low risk of cardiovascular disease

Heavy metals (arsenic, cadmium, lead, mercury) – elements that possess metallic properties and have a gravity measurement greater than 5.0

Hemorrhage – abnormal or excessive bleeding

Herbal therapy – herbal combination of tinctures, extracts and capsules used for cleansing and healing

Histamine – chemical released by the immune system that has potential negative effects on the body

Homeopathy – alternative medicines using herbs, natural substances to strengthen the immune system

Hormone – vital substances produced by the body that regulates many biological processes

Host – an organism on which another invading organism thrives on and obtains nourishment from

Human Growth Hormone (HGH) – a hormone that stimulates cell reproduction and growth, commonly seen as the normal increase in height through childhood; taken as a supplement HGH may increase muscle size but not necessarily muscle strength or performance

Hyaluronic acid – an organic substance that is regarded as the most effective natural skin moisturizer

Hydrochloric acid (HCL) – a strong corrosive stomach acid that helps digestion

Hydrogenation – process by which hydrogen atoms are combined with oil molecules to turn liquid oils into solids, destroying the nutritional value of the oil

Hypoallergenic – having a low capacity for being affected by allergies

I

Immune system – a complex system of organs, cells and proteins that protect the body against disease

Immunity – the body's ability to resist disease or infection

Infection – destructive invasion of body tissue by bacterial, fungal, viral or parasitic organisms

Infestation – destructive invasion of the body by worms, insects or protozoa

Inorganic – substances that do not contain carbon

Insulin – an anabolic hormone produced by the pancreas that regulates proper blood sugar levels

Intestinal flora – friendly bacteria in the digestive tract that are essential for digestion and metabolism

Isoflavones – a class of phytonutrients that protect against estrogen-based cancers like breast cancer

International unit (IU) – a measurement of a substance's potency, regardless of weight or volume

K

Kefir – fermented milk product that has anti-aging properties

Ketosis – a process of metabolism where the liver converts fats into fatty acids and is used for energy

Ketones – substances produced by the body as it breakdowns fats for energy

Kombucha – a sweetened fermented tea beverage that has detoxifying effects and healing properties

L

Lactase – an enzyme that converts lactose into glucose and is necessary for digesting milk and dairy

Lactic acid – an acid created from glucose metabolism that accumulates in the body after strenuous exercise causing muscle fatigue and pain

Lactobacilli – a species of bacteria that are able to convert lactose into lactic acid

Lactose – term referring to milk sugar

Lauric acid – a fatty acid found in coconut and palm kernel oil that has antimicrobial properties

LDL cholesterol (low density lipoprotein) – known as *bad cholesterol* that may cause cardiovascular disease

Lecithin – dark yellow fatty substances of which all living cell membranes are composed of

Legumes – seed pod that splits both sides when ripe (alfalfa, beans, carob, lentils, peanuts, peas, soy)

Lentils – a leguminous, climbing-vine plant containing only 2 seeds to a pod (beluga, black, green, red, white, yellow)

Liminoids – phytonutrients found in citrus fruits that help inhibit the production of cancer cells and HIV protease activity

Linolenic acid (LA) – an omega-6 essential fatty acid found in corn oil, safflower and sunflower oil

Lipids – natural substances that are soluble in the same solvents as fats and oils

Lipolysis – **r**efers to the chemical breakdown of body fat by enzymes that produce energy

Lipoprotein – protein molecule that helps transport fats around the bloodstream

Lipotropic – substances that help break down fat during metabolism and manage blood sugar levels

Lutein – phytonutrient that helps protect against macular degeneration (spinach, kale, turnip greens)

Lycopene – a phytonutrient that helps protect against prostate cancer and ultraviolet rays from the sun found in guava, pink grapefruit, tomatoes and watermelon

Lymph – a coagulable fluid created by blood plasma that circulates through the body to nourish cells

Lymph nodes – organs in the lymphatic system that filter and remove foreign substances

M

Macrobiotics – referring to a branch of Eastern medicine that uses grain as a staple food, and balances Yin (negative) and Yang (positive) foods together to overcome health issues

Macronutrients (proteins, carbohydrates and fats) – essential elements needed in large quantities to sustain proper health

Malabsorption – the inability to absorb nutrients from the intestines into the bloodstream

Melanoma – a rare type of skin cancer where a malignant tumor forms under the skin

Metabolic rate – refers to the rate the body converts food into energy, which is determined by calorie intake, muscle mass and exercise

Metabolism – process by which cells absorb nutrition and change food into energy

Mineral – naturally occurring substance that is essential for human life and vital to metabolic processes

Monoterpenes – phytonutrients that are the main constituent of essential oils and help protect the immune system

Monounsaturated fats (canola, olive, peanut and sunflower oils) – fatty acids that are not saturated with hydrogen, typically liquid at room temperature but will solidify when refrigerated

Mucus membranes – a lipid bi-layer of cells that line the cavities of the body that are involved with absorption, secretion and breathing

N

Naturopathy – alternative form of medicine using a combination of natural methods to combat disease and maintain health

Neurological disorder – a nervous system disorder that is marked by chemical or electrical abnormalities in the brain, spinal cord or the nerves connecting them (Alzheimer's disease, dementia, epilepsy, migraines, multiple sclerosis, Parkinson's disease, schizophrenia, sleep disorders etc.)

Nonessential Amino Acids – amino acids that can be produced by the body from other amino acids, therefore not essential to the human diet

Nutrient – a natural substance that all living organisms need for growth and survival

Nutrition – the science of turning food into fuel for the body to use

O

Organic – referring to foods that are grown naturally, without the use of synthetic chemicals like herbicides, pesticides or hormones

Osteoarthritis (OA) – also known as degenerative joint disease, it is the most common form of arthritis affecting approximately 90% of arthritis sufferers, characterized by cartilage degeneration, joint pain and inflammation, usually affecting larger joints (knees, hips, sometimes hands), associated with the wear & tear of aging, repetitive use and gradual onset of pain, may also cause bone spurs

Oxalates (oxalic acid) – organic substances found in humans, plants and animals of which high concentrations may lead to kidney stones; (oxalic acid foods include: amaranth, beans, beet greens, beer, berries, celery, chocolate, figs, kale, kiwi, leeks, nuts/seeds, okra, parsley, plums, quinoa, rhubarb, soy foods, spinach, squash, Swiss chard, tangerines, watercress, wheat germ)

Oxidation – chemical interactions between oxygen and other substances causing cellular decomposition and the production of free radicals

P

Parasite – a smaller organism living on/inside of a larger host, it is completely dependent on its host for nourishment and can be potentially damaging

Pepsin – a digestive enzyme released by the stomach to break down food proteins into peptides

Peptide – a compound made up of two or more amino acids that are broken down by protein molecules

pH (potential of hydrogen) – a measurement of the acidity and alkalinity of a substance or solution

Photosynthesis – the synthesis of organic compounds from inorganic compounds by plants and algae involving light energy

Phytonutrients – natural substances found in fruits and vegetables that protect the body against disease (chlorophyll, carotenoids, flavonoids, isoflavones, inositol, lignans, indoles, phenols, sulfides, terpenes)

Placebo – a preparation of pharmacologically inactive substances used in experimental comparisons of active substances

Plaque – a harmful substance that collects on brain tissue, inside the arteries and mouth and is believed to be associated with causing Alzheimer's disease

Pollutant – a toxic chemical which reduces the quality of the environment

Pollution – the presence of one or more pollutants in the environment

Polyphenols – a group of compounds found in plants that have at least one phenol unit per molecule

Polyps – rounded tissues bulging from the surface of an organ

Polysaccharides – a class of carbohydrates which breaks down during hydrolysis to a monosaccharide

Probiotics – substances that promote the growth of friendly bacteria in the body

Protein – nitrogen-based organic compounds made from amino acids that are the basic components of animal and vegetable tissues, needed for growth and repair

Proteolytic enzymes – enzymes that break down proteins and reduce the risk of cancer

Purines – natural substances that are part of the chemical structure of human, plant and animal genes, high concentrations may lead to arthritis, gout and inflammation (purine-rich foods include: anchovies, asparagus, bacon, beef, cauliflower, chicken, eggs, ham, herring, mackerel, mushrooms, mussels, oatmeal, organ meats, peas, pork, sardines, shellfish, smelt, spinach, sweetbreads, turkey, yeast),

R

RDA (Recommended Daily Allowance) – the basic amount of nutrients that should be consumed daily to maintain proper health

Reflexology – the practice of massaging/applying pressure to reflex points in the hands and feet that correspond to certain organs, glands and parts of the body encouraging therapeutic effects

Remission – the reversal of disease symptoms usually associated with cancer and multiple sclerosis

Respiratory tract – body structures that mediate the movement of air into and out of the body, like the airways, lungs and the respiratory muscles

Retinoic acid – the acid from vitamin A

Retrovirus – a type of virus that copies its RNA into the DNA of infected cells, manipulates its genetic function and begins replicating as part of the cell's DNA, suspected of causing leukemia and lymphoma

Rheumatoid Arthritis (RA) – far less common that osteoarthritis affecting about 10% of those with arthritis, abnormal autoimmune response characterized by inflammation of tissues that cover the joints causing redness, swelling and tenderness, usually affecting smaller joints (hands, wrists, ankles, feet) and organs (heart, kidneys, lungs), associated with prolonged morning stiffness exceeding 30 minutes, fatigue & fever, much more common among women

S

Saliva – a mixture of water, protein and salts that makes food easy to swallow and digest

Saturated fat (butter, chocolate, dairy, lard, meat) – regarded as unhealthy fat, it is typically solid at room temperature and has been shown to raise cholesterol levels

Saturation – term referring to fat molecules that cannot incorporate any more hydrogen atoms

Secretin – a hormone that causes the liver to make bile, the stomach to make pepsin and the pancreas to make digestive juices

Serotonin – a neurotransmitter in the brain essential for concentration, relaxation and sleep

Simple carbohydrate – a carbohydrate that is quickly digested and absorbed into the bloodstream

Stevia – a natural herbal sweetener native to South America that is much sweeter that sugar

Stress hormones (adrenaline, cortisol, DHEA, norepinephrine) – substance released by the body during times of stress

Sucrose – table sugar

Susceptibility – being predisposed, sensitive or at high risk of becoming infected by a disease

Symptom – an indication of an illness, disease or a change in normal function and well being

Synergy – the harmonious interaction between two or more substances where their combined ability is greater than their individual actions

Systemic – a term referring to the entire body system

T

T cell – a type of white blood cell with a special T cell receptor on the cell's surface that is an essential part of the immune system

Thermogenics – dietary supplements that increase metabolism and generate heat

Thyroid gland – internal thermostat regulating body temperature by secreting hormones that control energy used and calories burned

Tolerance – the capability of an organism to endure an unfavorable environment

Toxin – a poison that impairs health and bodily functions

Trace element – mineral required by the body in minute quantities for proper growth and development

Trans-fat – unsaturated fat produced through hydrogenation; increases risk of cardiovascular disease

Tremor – unintentional trembling or muscle movement of the body

Triglyceride – compound made up of three fatty acids and glycerol and is how fat is stored in the body

Tumor – an abnormal growth or mass of tissue that has the potential to become cancerous

U

Unsaturated fat (olive, flaxseed, safflower and fish oils) – known as healthy fat, these help reduce cholesterol and triglycerides levels in the blood

V

Vascular – term referring to the circulatory system

Vein – a blood vessel that returns blood from the body tissues back to the heart

Virus – an infectious agent that causes damage to its infected host and are not affected by antibiotics

Vitamin – organic substance obtained through diet to maintain proper health and support many biological functions

W

Water-soluble – the ability to dissolve in water

White blood cell – a blood cell that fights infection and repairs wounds

X

Xylitol – a natural sweetener made from birch bark that has antifungal properties, has a low glycemic index (GI) score and alkalizes the body

Y

Yang (heat, light and dryness) – one of two essential principles of Chinese medicine needed to create balance and harmony in the body, organs include the gallbladder, spleen, intestines and skin

Yin (cold, shadow and moisture) – the other essential principle of Chinese medicine needed to create balance and harmony in the body, organs include the liver, heart, kidneys, lungs and bones

Z

Zeaxanthin – a phytonutrient that protects against macular degeneration found in citrus fruits, eggs and green vegetables

~ List of References ~

*Anderson, Jean E. M.S., Deskins, Barbara Ph.D. *The Nutrition Bible – A Comprehensive No-Nonsense Guide to Foods, Nutrients, Additives, Preservatives, Pollutants and Everything Else We Eat and Drink.* New York, NY: HarperCollins Publishers, 1997

*Balch, Phyllis A., CNC. *Prescription for Nutritional Healing, 5th edition.* New York, NY: Penguin Group (Avery), 2010

*Beck, Leslie R.D. *Leslie Beck's Nutrition Encyclopedia.* Toronto, Ontario: Penguin Group, 2003

*Campbell, T. Colin, Ph.D., and Campbell, Thomas M. *The China Study – Startling Implications for Diet, Weight Loss and Long-term Health.* Dallas, TX: BenBella Books, 2005

*Chmelik, Stefan. *Chinese Herbal Secrets – The Key to Total Health.* New York, NY: The Ivy Press Limited, 1999

*Colbert, Don M.D. *Toxic Relief – Restore Health and Energy Through Fasting and Detoxification.* Lake Mary, FL: Siloam Press, 2003

*Duff, Roberta Larsen M.S., R.D. *American Diabetes Association Complete Food & Nutrition guide.* Hoboken, NJ: John Wiley & Sons Inc., 2006

*Kirschmann, Gayla J. and Kirschmann, John D. *Nutrition Almanac, 4th edition.* New York, NY: McGraw-Hill, 1996

*Liponis, Mark M.D. *Ultra Longevity – The Seven-Step Program for a Younger Healthier You.* New York, NY: Little, Brown and Company, 2008

*Mihesuah, Devon A., *Recovering Our Ancestors' Gardens – Indigenous Recipes and Guide to Diet and Fitness.* Lincoln, NB: University of Nebraska Press, 2005

*Miller, David Niven. *Grow Youthful – A Practical Guide to Slowing Your Aging.* Cottesloe, West Australia: John Hunt Publishing & O-Books, 2007

*Murray, Michael N.D. and Pizzorno, Joseph N.D. with Pizzorno, Lara M.A., L.M.T. *The Encyclopedia of Healing Foods.* New York, NY: Atria Books, 2005

*Plasker, Eric D.C. *The 100 Year Lifestyle.* Avon, MA: Adams Media Publishing, 2007

*Price, Weston A., D.D.S. *Nutrition and Physical Degeneration, 8th edition.* San Diego, CA: Price-Pottenger Nutrition Foundation, 2008

*Roizen, Michael F., M.D. and Oz, Mehmet C., M.D. *You Staying Young – The Owners Manual for Extending Your Warranty.* New York, NY: Free Press, 2007

*Somer, Elizabeth M.A., R.D. *Food & Mood – The Complete Guide to Eating Well and Feeling Your Best, 2nd edition.* New York, NY: Owl Books, 1999

*Tessmer, Kimberly A. R.D., L.D. *The Everything Nutrition Book – Boost Energy, Prevent Illness and Live Longer.* Avon, MA: Adams Media, 2003

*Trattler, Ross N.D., D.O. and Jones, Adrian N.D. *Better Health Through Natural Healing, 2nd edition.* Heatherton VIC, Australia: Hinkler Books, 2001

*Trowell, Hubert C. and Burkitt, Denis P. *Western Diseases: Their Emergence and Prevention.* Cambridge, MA: Harvard University Press, 1981

*Willcox, Bradley J. M.D., M.S., Willcox, Craig Ph.D., M.H.sc., and Suzuki, Makoto M.D., Ph.D. *The Okinawa Diet Plan –*

Get Leaner, Live Longer and Never Feel Hungry. New York, NY: Three Rivers Press, 2004

*Willcox, Bradley J. M.D., M.S., Willcox, Craig Ph.D., M.H.sc., Suzuki, Makoto M.D., Ph.D. *The Okinawa Program – How the World's Longest-lived People Achieve Everlasting Health-and how you can too.* New York, NY: Three Rivers Press, 2001

*Wilson, Dr. Lawrence. *Legal Guidelines for Unlicensed Practitioners.* Prescott, AZ: L.D. Wilson Consultants, 2007

*Yeager, Selene. *The Doctor's Book of Food Remedies.* Emmaus, PA: Rodale Press Inc., 2000

Permission to use the Optimal Health Food Pyramid granted by Dr. Michael T. Murray, N.D, Chairman, Dr. Murray Natural Living, Inc., DoctorMurray.com

Permission to use the Okinawa Diet Food Pyramid granted by Randall Willcox, Webmaster, Okinawa-Diet.com

Permission to use the Traditional Healthy Asian & Mediterranean Diet Pyramids granted by Birthe Creutz, Director of Finance and License Manager, Oldways Preservation & Exchange Trust, Oldwayspt.org

~ Resourceful Websites ~

Administration on Aging (AOA) – www.aoa.gov

Alzheimer's Association – www.alz.org

American Cancer Society (ACS) – www.cancer.org

American Diabetes Association (ADA) – www.diabetes.org

American Heart Association (AHA) – www.americanheart.org

American Institute for Cancer Research (AICR) – www.aicr.org

American Parkinson's Disease Association (APDA) – www.apdaparkinson.org

American Society for Nutrition (ASN) – www.nutrition.org

Arthritis Foundation – www.arthritis.org

California Certified Organic Farmers (CCOF) – www.ccof.org

Cancer Cure Foundation – www.cancure.org

Celiac Disease Center-University of Chicago – www.celiacdisease.net

Celiac Disease Foundation (CDF) – www.celiac.org

Center for Nutrition Policy and Promotion (CNPP) – www.cnpp.usda.gov/dietaryguidelines.htm

Crohn's and Colitis Foundation of America (CCFA) – www.ccfa.org

Cystic Fibrosis Foundation (CFF) – www.cff.org

Department of Health and Human Services (DHHS) – www.hhs.gov

Earthbound Farm – www.mypyramid.gov

Eating Right Pyramid – www.mypyramid.gov

Ecological Farming Association (EcoFarm) – www.eco-farm.org

Environmental Protection Agency (EPA) – www.epa.gov

Environmental Work Group (EWG) – www.ewg.org

EWG's 2010 Shoppers Guide to Pesticides – www.foodnews.org

Epilepsy Foundation of America – www.epilepsyfoundation.org

Food and Drug Administration (FDA) – www.fda.gov

Food Timeline – www.foodtimeline.org

Glycemic Index Foundation – www.glycemicindex.com

Hippocrates Health Institute (HHI) – www.hippocratesinst.org

Immune Deficiency Foundation (IDF) – www.primaryimmune.org

Institute of Medicine - Food and Nutrition Board (FNB) – www.iom.edu

International Federation of Organic Agricultural Movements (IFOAM) – www.ifoam.org

International Fitness Professionals Association (IFPA) – www.ifpa-fitness.com

Lance Armstrong Foundation (LAF) – www.livestrong.com

Leukemia and Lymphoma Society – www.leukemia-lymphoma.org

Linus Pauling Institute-Oregon State University – www.lpi.oregonstate.edu

Local Harvest – www.localharvest.org

Lupus Foundation of America (LFA) – www.lupus.org

Mayo Clinic – www.mayoclinic.com

Mental Health America (MHA) – www.nmha.org

Multiple Sclerosis Foundation (MSF) – www.msfacts.org

National Academy of Sciences (NAS) – www.nationalacademies.org

National Cancer Institute (NCI) – www.cancer.gov

National Center for Complimentary and Alternative Medicine (NCCAM) – www.nccam.nih.gov

National Council on Aging (NCOA) – www.ncoa.org

National Council on Alcoholism and Drug Dependence (NCADD) – www.ncadd.org

National Heart, Lung and Blood Institute (NHLBI) – www.nhlbi.nih.gov

National Sustainable Agriculture Information Service – www.attra.ncat.org

Natural Health Research Institute (NHRI) – www.naturalhealthresearch.org

National Kidney Foundation (NKF) – www.kidney.org

National Osteoporosis Foundation (NOF) – www.nof.org

National Parkinson Foundation (NPF) – www.parkinson.org

National Pesticide Information Center (NPIC) – www.npic.orst.edu

NSF International (The Public Health & Safety Company) – www.nsf.org

Oasis Advanced Wellness – www.oasisadvancedwellness.com

Okinawa Centenarian Study (OCS) – www.okicent.org

Okinawa Diet Program – www.okinawa-diet.com

Okinawa Research Center for Longevity Science (ORCLS) – www.orcls.org

Oldways Preservation & Exchange Trust – www.oldwayspt.org

Organic Consumers Association (OCA) – www.organicconsumers.org

Organic Farming Research Foundation (OFRF) – www.ofrf.org

Organic Trade Association (OTA) – www.ota.com

Organic Valley (co-op) – www.organicvalley.coop

Pacific Health Research and Education Institute (PHREI) – www.phrei.org

Parkinson's Institute – www.thepi.org

Price-Pottenger Nutrition Foundation (PPNF) – www.ppnf.org

School of Molecular Bioscience-University of Sydney – www.sydney.edu.au

Skin Cancer Foundation – www.skincancer.org

Traditional Chinese Medicine (TCM) – www.chinesemedicineherbs.net

United States Department of Agriculture (USDA) – www.usda.gov

Water Quality Association (WQA) – www.wqa.org

Weston A. Price Foundation – www.westonaprice.org

World Wide Opportunities on Organic Farms USA (WWOOF-USA) – www.wwoofusa.org

Organic Farming Organizations	
California Certified Organic Farmers (CCOF) 2155 Delaware Ave # 150 Santa Cruz, CA 95060-5732 (831) 423-2263 www.ccof.org	non-profit organic certification association that promotes organic agriculture, one of the first organizations to certify organic farms in North America, worked to legally define the term "organic", set guidelines for organic standards
Ecological Farming Association (EcoFarm) 2901 Park Avenue, Suite D-2 Soquel, CA 95073 (831) 763-2111 www.eco-farm.org	non-profit organization that promotes ecologically sound agriculture, sponsors educational events and answers questions from consumers, farmers and government agencies all over the United States
Hawaii Organic Farmers Association (HOFA) PO Box 6863 Hilo HI 96720 Phone: (808) 969-7789 www.hawaiiorganic.org	promotes organic farming practices, offers organic education and certifications in Hawaii, hosts training events, and publish a quarterly newsletter called "Rural Connections"
International Federation of Organic Agricultural Movements (IFOAM) Charles-de-Gaulle-Str. 5 53113 Bonn - Germany www.ifoam.org	worldwide organization that promotes organic farming practices in developing countries. IFOAM Organic Guarantee System (OGS) provides a uniform system of standards, quality verification and market guarantees for international organic integrity
Organic Farming Research Foundation (OFRF) 303 Potrero St., Ste. 29-203 Santa Cruz, CA 95060 (831) 426-6606 www.ofrf.org	non-profit organization that sponsors research of organic farming practices, educates the public and key decision-makers about current organic farming issues and communicates research results to farmers and growers interested in organic farming
World Wide Opportunities on Organic Farms USA (WWOOF-USA) 430 Forest Avenue Laguna Beach, CA 92651 (949) 715-9500 www.wwoofusa.org	international movement and information exchange sharing sustainable organic living practices, offers food, accommodations and learning opportunities in exchange for volunteer assistance
Local Harvest PO Box 1292 Santa Cruz, CA 95061 (831) 515-5602 www.localharvest.org	great resource for locating famer's markets, family farms and locally-grown organic produce by zip code, most comprehensive listing of Communities Supported Agriculture (CSA) Farms
Organic Valley (CROPP Cooperative) One Organic Way LaFarge, WI 54639 (608) 625-3025 www.organicvalley.coop	largest co-op of organic farmers in the U.S. and one of the leaders in organic agriculture, they support farm diversity and economic stability through organic farming practices and provide high-quality, organic-certified food products

~ About the Author ~

Rory M. Celmin is certified in sports nutrition from the International Fitness Professional Association (IFPA), received a Bachelor's Degree in English from California State University San Marcos (CSUSM) and has studied health and nutrition for over 25 years. His love of nutrition and preventative health is piqued traveling abroad, discovering unique nutritional solutions through a variety of organic foods and natural supplements. In his spare time he enjoys tennis, basketball, surfing, hiking and photography, and resides in sunny California.

@VitalityHealth9

Made in the USA
Monee, IL
12 September 2026

62980999R00114